CW00394841

THE ALL-IN-ONE PERIMENOPAUSE DIET FOR BEGINNERS

The Complete Nutritional Guide for Women in the 40's and 50's | Includes 100+ Wholesome Recipes

Ashley Brooke M.D.

COPYRIGHT

No part of this publication may be reproduced, stored in a retrieval system, transmitted, or distributed in any form or by any means, electronic, mechanical, photocopying, recording, scanning, or otherwise, without the prior written permission of the Publisher or authorization by payment of the appropriate per-copy fee to the Copyright, except as provided in Sections 107 or 108 of the United States Copyright Act of 1976.

Any and all implied guarantees of merchantability and fitness for a particular purpose are specifically disclaimed by both the publisher and the author. They have worked hard to ensure the information shown here is accurate, but they make no promises as to its completeness or accuracy. No guarantees are extended or constituted by any statements made by sales employees, either verbally or in writing.

It is recommended that you seek the advice of a professional whenever feasible, as the information and solutions provided here may not apply to your unique situation. Lost earnings, lost money, missed chances, and other comparable outcomes are not considered economic losses for which the publisher or author can be held accountable. It is important to remember that the electronic versions may exclude certain information that appeared in the print versions.

All rights reserved. Unauthorized use, reproduction, or distribution of this material is strictly prohibited and may result in legal action.

Table of Contents

CHAPTER 1: INTRODUCTION

You've found the full approach to supporting your heart health with the Perimenopause Diet for Heart Health cookbook. Hormonal changes occur during perimenopause, the time just before menopause begins, and these changes can have an effect on cardiovascular health. During this time of transition, women's cardiovascular health can be greatly aided by adopting a heart-healthy lifestyle and a nutritious diet.

Hormonal changes, especially a drop in estrogen levels, may have an effect on heart health during perimenopause. As estrogen levels naturally fall during perimenopause, women may be at a higher risk of developing cardiovascular disease. Women can reduce their vulnerability to cardiovascular disease by adopting a heart-healthy diet and way of life.

This cookbook is designed specifically for women in perimenopause, and it has a wide variety of heart-healthy foods and nutritional suggestions. Our goal is to equip you with information and tasty heart-healthy meals that won't sacrifice your enjoyment of life. Each dish was created with the intention of starting you on the path to a heart-healthy lifestyle, from the nutrient-dense ingredients to the heart-friendly cooking techniques.

Come along on our gastronomic journey as we investigate the role of diet in perimenopausal heart health. Let's take care of our hearts as a group so that we may face this pivotal time in our lives with energy, optimism, and a will to maintain our cardiovascular health for the rest of our lives. If you're ready to put your heart's health first and adopt a heart-healthy lifestyle, the "Perimenopause Diet for Heart Health" cookbook will be a reliable friend.

What is Perimenopause Diet for Heart Health?

The Perimenopause Diet for Heart Health is an eating plan designed to promote cardiovascular health in the years leading up to menopause. The fall in estrogen levels characteristic of perimenopause is one factor that can affect cardiovascular health. Perimenopause is associated with a decline in estrogen, which has a protective role in preventing cardiovascular disease and may raise the risk of cardiovascular problems. Therefore, at this time, it is very important to adopt a heart-healthy diet in order to reduce risks and improve overall heart health.

The Perimenopause Diet for Heart Health places an emphasis on consuming nutrient-rich foods that are beneficial to cardiovascular health and can help improve performance during this transitional period. Fiber, omega-3 fatty acids, antioxidants, potassium, and magnesium are just some of the heart-healthy elements that are promoted by this diet. Reduce inflammation, promote blood vessel function, and regulate blood pressure and cholesterol levels are just a few of the many ways these nutrients help keep your heart healthy.

Fruits, vegetables, whole grains, lean meats, and healthy fats are all encouraged on the diet. It recommends cutting back on meals that are bad for your heart, such those with added salt, refined sugar, and saturated and trans fats. Eating whole, unprocessed meals is the best way to provide your body the nutrients it needs to maintain healthy cardiovascular function and general health.

The Perimenopause Diet for Heart Health stresses not only what you eat, but how much of it, and how you consume it. Maintaining a healthy weight through portion management eases cardiovascular stress. Overeating may be avoided and a healthy connection with food can be fostered via the practice of mindful eating.

Constant water intake is also an important part of this diet. Maintaining a healthy blood volume and circulation is essential to heart health, which is why being hydrated is so important.

In addition to a heart-healthy diet, regular exercise is a cornerstone of the perimenopause phase. In order to strengthen the heart, enhance circulation, and promote overall cardiovascular function, regular physical activity, including both aerobic workouts and strength training, is essential.

The Perimenopause Diet for Heart Health is not a cookie-cutter plan of action. If you want specialized advice and assurance that your diet is in line with your health objectives and preferences, go to a licensed dietitian or healthcare expert.

The Perimenopause Diet for Heart Health is a preventative strategy for maintaining cardiovascular health at this pivotal time in a woman's life. Maintaining cardiovascular health and general vigor during perimenopause and beyond is possible for women who eat a balanced, nutrient-rich diet.

Perimenopause and Cardiovascular Risk

Hormonal changes occur during perimenopause as a woman's body gets ready for menopause, making this a pivotal time in her life. Estrogen levels vary and its fall may affect cardiovascular health at this time of transition. Estrogen aids in the prevention of cardiovascular disease and the control of cholesterol levels. During perimenopause, estrogen levels drop, which increases the risk of certain cardiovascular risk factors.

Changes in lipid profile, including elevation of low-density lipoprotein ("bad") cholesterol and reduction of high-density lipoprotein ("good") cholesterol, are a major cause for alarm during perimenopause. Plaque in the arteries, caused by high levels of LDL cholesterol, can increase the risk of atherosclerosis and cardiovascular disease. Decreased levels of good cholesterol (HDL) also make the heart less protected, increasing the danger of cardiovascular disease.

It's also possible that insulin sensitivity shifts during perimenopause, raising the likelihood of insulin resistance and, ultimately, type 2 diabetes. Obesity, hypertension, and abnormal lipid profiles are all cardiovascular risk factors that can be exacerbated by insulin resistance.

Blood pressure is another potential change during perimenopause that might impact cardiovascular risk. Higher blood pressure, which can strain the heart and raise the risk of heart disease, may be a result of fluctuating hormone levels.

During perimenopause, cardiovascular risk can also be affected by changes in nutrition, physical exercise, and stress levels. The risks associated with being overweight can be exacerbated by making unhealthy food choices and not getting enough exercise. Emotional eating and smoking are two harmful ways people deal with stress that can have a negative effect on cardiovascular health.

Although perimenopause is a time of increased cardiovascular risk, it is nevertheless a crucial time for women to take care of their heart health. Women can reduce the effects of hormonal shifts on their cardiovascular risk factors by adopting a heart-healthy lifestyle, which includes a balanced diet, frequent exercise, stress management strategies, and, if necessary, suitable medicines. Heart health may be monitored and treated promptly with the aid of frequent checkups and discussions with medical specialists. Women's heart health and well-being can benefit from having more information and resources available to them when they enter the perimenopause.

Common Heart Health Challenges in Hormonal Changes

Several prevalent issues with women's heart health are associated with hormonal changes, especially during perimenopause and menopause. The cardiovascular system is vulnerable to the effects of fluctuating estrogen levels and the risk factors they add.

Changes in lipid profiles pose a significant threat to cardiovascular health during periods of hormonal transition. Estrogen protects against the detrimental effects of excessive cholesterol by boosting high-density lipoprotein (HDL), or "good" cholesterol, and reducing low-density lipoprotein (LDL), or "bad" cholesterol. When estrogen levels drop, bad cholesterol (LDL) tends to rise while good cholesterol (HDL) drops, which can raise the risk of atherosclerosis and cardiovascular disease.

Blood pressure management can be affected by hormonal shifts. Vasodilatory effects of estrogen include relaxing and widening blood vessels, both of which contribute to reduced blood pressure. Lower estrogen levels have been linked to less flexible blood arteries and an increase in blood pressure. Heart disease, heart attacks, and strokes are all risks that rise with elevated blood pressure.

Hormonal fluctuations, especially during perimenopause and menopause, often result in an increase in body weight and a shift in overall body composition. Abdominal fat gain is particularly susceptible to hormonal influences. Visceral fat, often known as belly fat, is strongly linked to metabolic issues like insulin resistance and heart disease.

Insulin resistance and glucose metabolism are both susceptible to hormonal fluctuations. Women may be more at risk for developing type 2 diabetes and insulin resistance when estrogen levels decline. When combined with other risk factors, diabetes increases the likelihood of developing cardiovascular disease.

The endothelium is the lining of the blood vessels and its function can be affected by hormone fluctuations. Endothelial health is critical for avoiding atherosclerosis and keeping blood flowing freely. Endothelial dysfunction, which may contribute to the development of heart disease, may be exacerbated by low estrogen levels.

Maintaining cardiovascular health is dependent on addressing these issues during hormonal shifts. Hormonal shifts can be less detrimental to heart health if people adopt heart-healthy lifestyles, such as eating right, exercising regularly, managing stress, and not smoking or drinking to excess. The heart's health is crucial at this time of profound change, and regular checkups and discussions with healthcare specialists can give individualized guidance and actions to address particular risk factors. Better heart health and general wellbeing may be achieved by equipping women with information and proactive techniques as they deal with hormonal shifts and beyond.

CHAPTER 2: DIET FOR MAINTAINING A HEALTHY HEART

A healthy heart is essential to enjoying a full life, and a nutritious diet is a key factor in promoting cardiovascular wellness. Foods high in nutrients that have been shown to improve heart health and lower cardiovascular disease risk are the main emphasis of a diet designed to keep your ticker in good working order.

Fruits and vegetables should play a central role in your heart-healthy diet. Antioxidants, fiber, vitamins, and minerals may all be found in abundance in plant-based diets. Half your plate should be made up of bright fruits and vegetables since they are good for your heart and assist with things like blood pressure and inflammation.

A heart-healthy diet should also include plenty of whole grains. Brown rice, quinoa, oats, and whole wheat are just few of the whole grains that are high in fiber and can aid in lowering cholesterol and maintaining healthy blood sugar levels. Substituting healthy grains for processed ones might improve cardiovascular health and provide you more prolonged energy.

In order to keep your heart healthy, choose lean proteins like fish, chicken, beans, lentils, and tofu. Salmon, mackerel, and sardines, which are all rich in omega-3 fatty acids and hence decrease inflammation and lessen the risk of heart disease, are particularly beneficial. Fiber-rich and low in saturated fat, plant-based proteins like beans and lentils are good for your heart.

A heart-healthy diet must include these beneficial fats. Fats found in avocados, almonds, seeds, and olive oil are all good for you. Monounsaturated and polyunsaturated fats, which are plentiful in these oils, have been shown to reduce LDL cholesterol and, by extension, the risk of heart disease. These fats are high in calories, thus they should be consumed in moderation.

For the sake of your heart, it's important to reduce your intake of saturated fats, trans fats, and cholesterol. Saturated and trans fats are known to increase LDL cholesterol, whereas consuming too much dietary cholesterol has been linked to atherosclerotic plaque formation. The best way to control intake of these unhealthy fats is to consume less red meat, processed foods, and high-fat dairy.

Maintaining a healthy heart also requires cutting back on salt intake. Heavy blood pressure is a known risk factor for cardiovascular disease and may be exacerbated by a diet heavy in salt. Avoid processed and packaged foods as they typically contain excessive amounts of salt. Herbs and spices can be used in place of salt to add flavor to cuisine.

Finally, heart health depends on you drinking enough water. Keeping up a healthy blood volume and blood flow can be aided by drinking enough of water. Drinking less alcohol and fewer sugary drinks is also good for your heart.

Support cardiovascular health and lower the risk of cardiovascular disease by eating a heart-healthy diet rich in a wide range of fruits, vegetables, whole grains, lean meats, and healthy fats while limiting processed and high-sodium meals. When making dietary adjustments, it's important to talk to a doctor or a certified dietitian to get advice tailored to your specific condition and goals.

Key Nutrients for Heart Health

There are a number of essential nutrients that help maintain heart health and lower the risk of cardiovascular disease. Consuming foods rich in these nutrients has been shown to improve cardiovascular health and cardiovascular function.

Eicosapentaenoic acid (EPA) and docosahexaenoic acid (DHA) are two examples of omega-3 fatty acids that are particularly important for cardiovascular health. Plant sources such as chia seeds, flaxseeds, and walnuts, and animal ones such as salmon, mackerel, and sardines are all good places to look. Omega-3 fatty acids are beneficial for the heart because they help lower inflammation, triglyceride levels, and general heart health.

Fruits, vegetables, whole grains, legumes, and nuts are excellent sources of the dietary fiber that is so important to keeping your heart healthy. In particular, soluble fiber aids in reducing LDL cholesterol levels by eliminating it from the body after attaching to it in the digestive tract. The satiety brought on by eating high-fiber meals also aids in weight control and lowers the likelihood of developing obesity, which is a risk factor for cardiovascular disease.

The heart can be protected from the oxidative stress induced by free radicals thanks to antioxidants, which are abundant in fruits and vegetables of all hues. Inflammation is decreased, blood vessel function is enhanced, and general cardiovascular health is promoted by these effects. Berries, leafy greens, citrus fruits, and bell peppers are all excellent sources of antioxidants.

Potassium is essential for keeping blood pressure in a healthy range. It reduces the heart's workload by neutralizing sodium's effects. Bananas, sweet potatoes, spinach, avocados, and beans are some examples of foods that are rich in potassium.

Magnesium is essential for healthy heart function and is involved in hundreds of other biochemical activities in the body. It's beneficial for blood pressure, heart rate, and relaxing of blood vessels. Leafy greens, nuts, seeds, whole grains, and legumes are all excellent food sources.

Because of its involvement in calcium absorption and its aid in maintaining healthy blood vessel function, vitamin D is essential for heart health. Vitamin D deficiency has been linked to an increased risk of cardiovascular disease. Vitamin D may be obtained by exposure to sunshine, but it can also be obtained through diet from fortified foods, fatty fish, and egg yolks.

Vitamin K aids in clotting blood and is important for healthy arteries. Foods like broccoli, Brussels sprouts, and vegetable oils are good sources.

You may improve your heart health and lower your risk of cardiovascular disease by eating a diet high in these nutrients. The cornerstone of fostering optimum cardiac function and general well-being is a diet that is both varied and rich in whole foods. Although nutrition plays a significant role in promoting heart health, it is important to remember that other lifestyle variables, such as exercise, stress management, and not smoking, all play a role in ensuring optimal cardiovascular wellness. As always, it's best to go to a doctor or a nutritionist to get advice tailored to your specific health situation and objectives.

Incorporating Heart Friendly Recipes (foods to include for heart health)

Heart-healthy dishes may be a tasty and pleasurable method to improve one's cardiovascular health. You may make delicious meals that are also good for your heart by using foods high in nutrients that have been shown to have a preventive effect on the cardiovascular system.

Eat a bowl of oatmeal for breakfast, which is good for your heart, and top it with some berries and nuts or seeds. The soluble fiber in oats is beneficial because it reduces bad cholesterol (LDL). Berries' high concentration of heart-protective antioxidants pairs well with the beneficial fats and fiber found in nuts and seeds. Greek yogurt, a good source of both protein and calcium, is another option.

Try a salad for lunch, they're colorful and healthy. Greens like spinach or kale provide a great foundation for heart-healthy toppings like grilled chicken or salmon, avocado slices, cherry tomatoes, bell peppers, and more. The monounsaturated fats in avocado and the omega-3s in salmon make for a healthy diet. Olive oil, lemon juice, and a pinch of herbs make a simple vinaigrette that adds taste and heart-healthy lipids to your salad.

A stir-fry with quinoa and vegetables is a heart-healthy alternative for dinner. Quinoa is a complete protein and a great source of fiber, while the vibrant veggies provide a wide variety of nutrients, including vitamins, minerals, and antioxidants. Garlic, ginger, and low-sodium soy sauce are excellent additions to a vegetable stir-fry cooked in a tiny quantity of heart-healthy avocado oil.

Include fish in your weekly meal plan by cooking heart-healthy dishes like baked or grilled salmon. Omega-3 fatty acids, which are abundant in salmon, have been shown to have anti-inflammatory and pro-heart health effects. Salmon can be baked or grilled after being marinated in olive oil, lemon juice, and herbs.

Treat yourself to a heart-healthy dessert by making a delicious fruit salad. Fruits with a wide range of colors offer a wide range of health advantages, including high fiber and antioxidant content. Toss in some chopped nuts for texture and some heart-healthy fats.

Keep your heart healthy by drinking green or hibiscus tea all day long. Antioxidant-rich and linked to better heart health, these teas are a popular choice.

Portion control is key, as is minimizing the use of salt and added sugars in cooking. Baking, grilling, and steaming are all healthful alternatives to frying.

Avoid using too much salt and instead flavor your food using herbs and spices.

You can do wonders for your heart health and your taste buds by introducing heart-healthy foods into your diet. Eating a variety of whole, nutrient-dense foods is an excellent way to support your cardiovascular system and general health, and it can also be an enjoyable culinary adventure.

CHAPTER 3: MANAGING BLOOD PRESSURE

Controlling one's blood pressure is a crucial part of maintaining cardiovascular health and avoiding diseases of the heart and blood vessels. Hypertension, or high blood pressure, puts extra stress on the cardiovascular system and raises the risk of cardiovascular problems including heart attacks and strokes. Several therapies and adjustments in lifestyle can aid in keeping blood pressure in a healthy range.

Maintaining a healthy blood pressure can be accomplished in part by eating heart-friendly foods. Blood pressure can be lowered by eating a diet high in fruits, vegetables, whole grains, lean meats, and healthy fats. In particular, the DASH (Dietary

Approaches to Stop Hypertension) diet, which has been demonstrated to be helpful for lowering blood pressure, places an emphasis on these nutrient-dense foods. Too much salt in the diet can raise blood pressure, therefore cutting back is essential. Avoid processed and packaged foods as they typically contain excessive amounts of salt. Instead of adding salt to your food, try seasoning it with herbs and spices.

Getting regular exercise is also crucial for controlling blood pressure. Aerobic workouts, such as brisk walking, cycling, swimming, and dancing, have been shown to reduce blood pressure. Aim for at least 150 minutes of aerobic activity each week, split up into 75 minutes of moderate-intensity and 75 minutes of vigorous-intensity sessions. Weightlifting and other forms of strength training are also beneficial for helping keep blood pressure in check.

Controlling blood pressure is intricately tied to keeping a healthy weight. Dropping extra pounds, especially around the midsection, can have a dramatic effect on blood pressure. Maintaining a healthy weight and managing blood pressure both benefit from a combination of a heart-friendly diet and frequent exercise.

Maintaining a normal blood pressure reading requires regular stress management. Chronic stress can raise blood pressure, therefore it's important to find ways to de-stress on a regular basis. Relaxation and stress reduction can be achieved by practices such as deep breathing, meditation, yoga, and time spent in nature.

Controlling blood pressure also involves limiting alcohol intake. While some research suggests that drinking alcohol in moderation may be beneficial for heart health, heavy drinking is linked to an increase in blood pressure and an increased risk of cardiovascular disease. Women should consume no more than one alcoholic beverage every day, following the guidelines.

Medication may be recommended by a doctor if controlling blood pressure via lifestyle modifications alone proves insufficient. Medication for hypertension has been shown to be helpful in lowering blood pressure and avoiding problems. Taking prescription medicine as directed by your doctor is crucial.

Modifying one's lifestyle, learning to cope with stress, and, if required, taking medication are all components of blood pressure control. Supporting heart health, lowering the risk of cardiovascular disease, and improving general well-being are all possible outcomes from taking preventative measures to lower blood pressure. Visits to the doctor on a regular basis allow for the tracking of blood pressure and the implementation of any necessary actions to keep it at a healthy level.

Maintaining a Healthy Weight for Heart Health

Maintaining a healthy weight is a crucial aspect of promoting heart health and reducing the risk of cardiovascular disease. High blood pressure, elevated cholesterol levels, and insulin resistance are just a few of the medical issues that can result from carrying extra weight around the middle. People may take charge of their cardiovascular health by achieving and maintaining a healthy weight.

In order to maintain a healthy weight and heart, dietary changes must be made. Consuming a diet rich in fruits, vegetables, whole grains, lean meats, and healthy fats can help people feel full and fed without adding excess calories. Because of their links to obesity and cardiovascular disease, processed meals, sugary drinks, and foods rich in saturated and trans fats should be avoided.

Keeping up with a regular exercise routine is essential for both weight management and cardiovascular health. Aerobic activity, such brisk walking, running, cycling, or swimming, is an excellent way to become in shape and burn calories. Muscle mass, which may be increased by strength training activities like lifting weights or completing bodyweight exercises, might be helpful in managing weight.

Controlling one's portion sizes is essential for staying at a healthy weight. When consumed in excess, even nutritious meals can contribute to weight gain. Better food decisions may be made when people are aware of their bodies' hunger and fullness cues and practice mindful eating. For weight control, it's crucial to pay attention to serving amounts and avoid going overboard.

Maintaining a healthy weight depends on a number of factors, but one that is frequently forgotten is getting enough sleep. Hormonal imbalances brought on by sleep deprivation have been linked to increased hunger and a desire for junk food. Getting between 7 and 9 hours of excellent sleep nightly will help with many aspects of health, including maintaining a healthy weight.

Reducing stress is also important for keeping the pounds off. Emotional eating and making unhealthy food choices are two ways in which stress can contribute to weight gain. Meditation, yoga, deep breathing exercises, and time spent in nature are just a few examples of stress-reduction methods that can aid in weight control and help people deal with stress in a more constructive way.

Maintaining a healthy weight has several health benefits, especially for one's heart, and should be prioritized over aesthetic concerns. If you need to lose weight, it's usually better to do it slow and steady rather than resort to drastic tactics. Maintaining a healthy weight is beneficial for cardiovascular health and general vigor, and consulting with a healthcare provider or registered dietitian may give tailored direction and support in this endeavor. Maintaining a healthy weight and keeping tabs on other health indicators can aid folks on the path to better heart health.

CHAPTER 4: 100+ DELICIOUS PERIMENOPAUSE DIET RECIPES

BREAKFAST RECIPES YOU SHOULD TRY!

Oatmeal with Fresh Berries:

Ingredients

1/2 cup rolled oats

1 cup water or low-fat milk

Fresh berries (e.g., strawberries, blueberries, raspberries)

Honey (optional)

Instructions

In a saucepan, bring the water or milk to a boil.

Add the rolled oats and reduce the heat to low. Cook for about 5 minutes or until the oats are soft and creamy.

Remove from heat and transfer the oatmeal to a bowl.

Top with fresh berries and drizzle with honey, if desired.

Greek Yogurt Parfait:

Ingredients

1 cup Greek yogurt

1 ripe banana, sliced

Fresh strawberries, sliced

2 tablespoons granola

Instructions

In a glass or bowl, layer half of the Greek yogurt.

Add half of the sliced banana and strawberries on top of the yogurt.

Sprinkle 1 tablespoon of granola over the fruits.

Repeat the layering process with the remaining ingredients.

Chia Seed Pudding:

Ingredients

1/4 cup chia seeds

1 cup unsweetened almond milk

Fresh fruits (e.g., berries, kiwi, mango)

Instructions

In a jar or bowl, mix the chia seeds and almond milk thoroughly.

Refrigerate the mixture overnight or for at least 4 hours, stirring occasionally.

Before serving, top with fresh fruits of your choice.

Avocado Toast:

Ingredients

1 ripe avocado

2 slices of whole-grain bread

1 small tomato, sliced

Black pepper, to taste

Instructions

Cut the avocado in half, remove the pit, and scoop the flesh into a bowl.

Mash the avocado with a fork until it reaches your desired consistency.

Toast the bread slices until they are lightly browned and crispy.

Spread the mashed avocado evenly on each slice of toast.

Place the sliced tomatoes on top of the avocado and sprinkle with black pepper.

Spinach and Mushroom Omelette:

Ingredients

3 egg whites

Handful of fresh spinach leaves

1/4 cup sliced mushrooms

Salt and pepper to taste

Cooking spray or a teaspoon of olive oil

Instructions

In a bowl, whisk the egg whites and season with salt and pepper.

Heat a non-stick pan over medium heat and add cooking spray or olive oil.

Add the sliced mushrooms to the pan and sauté until they soften.

Add the fresh spinach leaves to the pan and cook until wilted.

Pour the whisked egg whites into the pan, making sure they cover the mushrooms and spinach evenly.

Cook until the omelette is set and the edges are lightly browned.

Fold the omelette in half and serve.

Quinoa Breakfast Bowl:

Ingredients

1/2 cup quinoa, rinsed

1 cup water or low-sodium vegetable broth

2 tablespoons sliced almonds

2 tablespoons chopped dates

Pinch of ground cinnamon

Instructions

In a saucepan, combine the quinoa and water or vegetable broth. Bring to a boil.

Reduce the heat to low, cover, and simmer for about 15 minutes or until the quinoa is cooked and the liquid is absorbed.

Fluff the quinoa with a fork and transfer it to a serving bowl.

Top the quinoa with sliced almonds, chopped dates, and a sprinkle of ground cinnamon.

Green Smoothie:

Ingredients

1 cup fresh spinach leaves

1 cup kale leaves, destemmed

1 ripe banana

1 cup unsweetened almond milk

Ice cubes (optional)

Instructions

In a blender, add the spinach, kale, banana, and almond milk.

Blend until the mixture reaches a smooth consistency.

If desired, add ice cubes and blend again until the smoothie is chilled.

Pour the green smoothie into a glass and serve.

Cottage Cheese with Pineapple:

Ingredients

1 cup low-fat cottage cheese

1 cup fresh pineapple chunks

Instructions

In a bowl, serve the low-fat cottage cheese.

Add the fresh pineapple chunks on top.

Whole Grain Pancakes:

Ingredients

1 cup whole grain flour

1 tablespoon baking powder

1/4 teaspoon salt

1 cup low-fat milk

1 large egg

1 tablespoon vegetable oil

Fresh berries for topping

Maple syrup (optional, for drizzling)

Instructions

In a large bowl, whisk together the whole grain flour, baking powder, and salt.

In a separate bowl, whisk together the low-fat milk, egg, and vegetable oil.

Pour the wet ingredients into the dry ingredients and stir until just combined.

Heat a non-stick pan or griddle over medium heat and lightly coat it with cooking spray or a little vegetable oil.

Pour 1/4 cup of the pancake batter onto the pan for each pancake.

Cook until bubbles form on the surface, then flip and cook the other side until golden brown.

Serve the whole grain pancakes with fresh berries on top and drizzle with maple syrup if desired.

Fruit Salad:

Ingredients

1 cup orange segments

1 cup apple slices

1 cup seedless grapes

1 cup diced mixed fruits (e.g., kiwi, berries, mango)

Fresh mint leaves for garnish (optional)

Instructions

In a large bowl, combine all the fruits.

Gently toss the fruits together until well mixed.

Garnish with fresh mint leaves if desired and serve.

Smoothie Bowl:

Ingredients

1 cup frozen mixed berries

1 ripe banana

1/2 cup unsweetened almond milk

1 tablespoon chia seeds

2 tablespoons sliced almonds

Fresh berries and coconut flakes for topping

Instructions

In a blender, combine the frozen mixed berries, banana, and almond milk.

Blend until the mixture reaches a thick and smooth consistency.

Pour the smoothie into a bowl.

Top the smoothie with chia seeds, sliced almonds, fresh berries, and coconut flakes.

Poached Eggs with Asparagus:

Ingredients

2 large eggs

8-10 asparagus spears, trimmed

Salt and pepper to taste

1 teaspoon white vinegar (optional)

Instructions

Fill a large saucepan with water and bring it to a simmer. If using vinegar, add it to the water.

Gently crack each egg into a small bowl or cup.

Create a gentle whirlpool in the simmering water and carefully slide one egg at a time into the center of the whirlpool.

Poach the eggs for about 3-4 minutes or until the whites are set but the yolks are still runny.

While the eggs are poaching, steam the asparagus spears until tender-crisp.

Remove the poached eggs from the water with a slotted spoon and place them on a plate lined with paper towels to drain excess water.

Serve the poached eggs with the steamed asparagus. Season with salt and pepper to taste.

Apple Cinnamon Overnight Oats:

Ingredients

1/2 cup rolled oats

1/2 cup unsweetened almond milk

1/2 cup diced apples

1 tablespoon chia seeds

1/2 teaspoon cinnamon

1 teaspoon honey or maple syrup (optional)

Instructions

In a jar or container, combine the rolled oats, almond milk, diced apples, chia seeds, and cinnamon.

Stir well to mix all the ingredients together.

Cover the jar and refrigerate overnight or for at least 4 hours.

In the morning, give the mixture a good stir.

If desired, drizzle with honey or maple syrup for sweetness.

Enjoy the apple cinnamon overnight oats cold or heat them up in the microwave before eating.

Breakfast Burrito:

Ingredients

2 large eggs

2 whole-grain tortillas

1/4 cup canned black beans, rinsed and drained

1/4 avocado, sliced

2 tablespoons salsa

Salt and pepper to taste

Cooking spray or a teaspoon of olive oil

Instructions

In a bowl, whisk the eggs and season with salt and pepper.

Heat a non-stick pan over medium heat and add cooking spray or olive oil.

Pour the whisked eggs into the pan and cook, stirring occasionally until scrambled and cooked through.

Warm the tortillas in a dry skillet or microwave.

Place half of the scrambled eggs on each tortilla.

Top with black beans, avocado slices, and salsa.

Roll up the tortillas, tucking in the sides as you go.

Serve the breakfast burritos warm.

Walnut and Banana Muffins:

Ingredients

1 1/2 cups whole wheat flour

1 teaspoon baking powder

1/2 teaspoon baking soda

1/4 teaspoon salt

1/2 teaspoon ground cinnamon

1/4 cup unsweetened applesauce

1/4 cup honey or maple syrup

1/4 cup unsweetened almond milk

2 ripe bananas, mashed

1/4 cup chopped walnuts

Instructions

Preheat the oven to 350°F (175°C) and line a muffin tin with paper liners.

In a large bowl, whisk together the whole wheat flour, baking powder, baking soda, salt, and ground cinnamon.

In a separate bowl, mix the applesauce, honey or maple syrup, almond milk, and mashed bananas.

Pour the wet ingredients into the dry ingredients and stir until just combined.

Fold in the chopped walnuts.

Divide the batter evenly among the muffin cups, filling each about 3/4 full.

Bake for 18-20 minutes or until a toothpick inserted into the center comes out clean.

Allow the muffins to cool in the pan for a few minutes, then transfer them to a wire rack to cool completely.

Blueberry Bran Muffins:

Ingredients

1 cup wheat bran

1 cup whole wheat flour

1 teaspoon baking powder

1/2 teaspoon baking soda

1/4 teaspoon salt

1/2 teaspoon ground cinnamon

1/4 cup unsweetened applesauce

1/4 cup honey or maple syrup

1/4 cup unsweetened almond milk

1 large egg

1 cup fresh or frozen blueberries

Instructions

Preheat the oven to 375°F (190°C) and line a muffin tin with paper liners.

In a bowl, combine the wheat bran, whole wheat flour, baking powder, baking soda, salt, and ground cinnamon.

In a separate bowl, mix the applesauce, honey or maple syrup, almond milk, and egg until well combined.

Add the wet ingredients to the dry ingredients and stir until just combined.

Gently fold in the blueberries.

Divide the batter evenly among the muffin cups, filling each about 3/4 full.

Bake for 15-18 minutes or until a toothpick inserted into the center comes out clean.

Allow the muffins to cool in the pan for a few minutes, then transfer them to a wire rack to cool completely.

Veggie Frittata:

Ingredients

4 large eggs

1/4 cup diced bell peppers (any color)

1/4 cup diced onions

1 cup fresh spinach leaves

1 tablespoon olive oil

Salt and pepper to taste

Instructions

Preheat the oven to 375°F (190°C).

In a bowl, whisk the eggs and season with salt and pepper.

In an oven-safe non-stick skillet, heat the olive oil over medium heat.

Add the diced bell peppers and onions to the skillet, and sauté until softened.

Add the fresh spinach leaves to the skillet and cook until wilted.

Pour the whisked eggs over the vegetables in the skillet, making sure they cover everything evenly.

Cook on the stovetop for a minute or until the edges start to set.

Transfer the skillet to the preheated oven and bake for about 10-12 minutes or until the frittata is fully set and lightly golden on top.

Remove from the oven and let it cool slightly before slicing and serving.

Peanut Butter Banana Smoothie:

Ingredients

1 ripe banana

1 cup low-fat milk (or almond milk for a dairy-free option)

1 tablespoon natural peanut butter

1 teaspoon honey (optional, for added sweetness)

Ice cubes (optional)

Instructions

In a blender, combine the ripe banana, low-fat milk, peanut butter, and honey (if using).

Blend until the smoothie reaches a creamy consistency.

If you prefer a thicker smoothie, add a few ice cubes and blend again until well mixed.

Pour the peanut butter banana smoothie into a glass and enjoy.

Breakfast Quinoa with Almonds:

Ingredients

1/2 cup quinoa, rinsed

1 cup low-fat milk (or water)

1/4 cup sliced almonds

1 teaspoon honey (optional, for sweetness)

Instructions

In a saucepan, combine the quinoa and low-fat milk (or water).

Bring the mixture to a boil, then reduce the heat to low.

Simmer for about 15 minutes or until the quinoa is cooked and the liquid is absorbed.

Fluff the quinoa with a fork and transfer it to a serving bowl.

Top the quinoa with sliced almonds and drizzle with honey if desired.

Acai Bowl:

Ingredients

1 packet frozen acai puree (unsweetened)

1 ripe banana

1/2 cup unsweetened almond milk (or any preferred milk)

Toppings: Granola, sliced strawberries, coconut flakes, chia seeds

Instructions

In a blender, combine the frozen acai puree, ripe banana, and unsweetened almond milk.

Blend until you achieve a thick and smooth consistency.

Pour the acai mixture into a bowl.

Top the acai bowl with granola, sliced strawberries, coconut flakes, and chia seeds.

Enjoy the acai bowl immediately.

LUNCH RECIPES YOU SHOULD TRY!

Grilled Chicken Salad:

Ingredients

2 boneless, skinless chicken breasts

6 cups mixed greens (lettuce, spinach, arugula, etc.)

1 cup cherry tomatoes, halved

1 cucumber, sliced

1/4 cup red onion, thinly sliced

1/4 cup balsamic vinaigrette dressing (store-bought or homemade)

Salt and pepper to taste

Olive oil for grilling

Instructions

Preheat your grill or stovetop grill pan over medium-high heat.

Season the chicken breasts with salt and pepper.

Lightly brush the grill with olive oil to prevent sticking.

Grill the chicken breasts for about 6-7 minutes per side or until cooked through and no longer pink in the center.

Remove the chicken from the grill and let it rest for a few minutes before slicing it into thin strips.

In a large bowl, combine the mixed greens, cherry tomatoes, cucumber, and red onion.

Add the grilled chicken strips on top.

Drizzle the balsamic vinaigrette dressing over the salad.

Toss the salad gently to coat everything with the dressing.

Divide the salad among serving plates and serve immediately.

Quinoa Stuffed Bell Peppers:

Ingredients

4 bell peppers (any color)

1 cup cooked quinoa

1 cup black beans (canned or cooked)

1 cup corn kernels (fresh, canned, or frozen)

1 avocado, diced

1/2 cup cherry tomatoes, halved

1/4 cup chopped cilantro

Juice of 1 lime

Salt and pepper to taste

Instructions

Preheat the oven to 375°F (190°C).

Cut the tops off the bell peppers and remove the seeds and membranes.

In a bowl, combine the cooked quinoa, black beans, corn, avocado, cherry tomatoes, cilantro, lime juice, salt, and pepper.

Stuff each bell pepper with the quinoa mixture.

Place the stuffed bell peppers in a baking dish and cover with foil.

Bake for about 25-30 minutes or until the peppers are tender.

Serve the quinoa stuffed bell peppers warm.

Baked Salmon with Steamed Broccoli:

Ingredients

2 salmon fillets

1 tablespoon olive oil

1 lemon, sliced

Salt and pepper to taste

2 cups broccoli florets

Instructions

Preheat the oven to 400°F (200°C).

Place the salmon fillets on a baking sheet lined with parchment paper.

Drizzle the olive oil over the salmon and season with salt and pepper.

Lay lemon slices on top of the salmon.

Bake the salmon for about 12-15 minutes or until it flakes easily with a fork.

While the salmon is baking, steam the broccoli until tender-crisp.

Serve the baked salmon with steamed broccoli on the side.

Chickpea and Vegetable Stir-Fry:

Ingredients

1 can (15 ounces) chickpeas, rinsed and drained

1 red bell pepper, sliced

1 yellow bell pepper, sliced

1 cup snow peas

1 cup broccoli florets

2 tablespoons low-sodium soy sauce

1 tablespoon hoisin sauce

1 tablespoon sesame oil

1 tablespoon minced ginger

2 cloves garlic, minced

2 green onions, sliced (for garnish)

Cooked brown rice or quinoa (optional, for serving)

Instructions

In a large skillet or wok, heat the sesame oil over medium-high heat.

Add the sliced bell peppers, snow peas, and broccoli to the skillet. Stir-fry for about 3-4 minutes until the vegetables start to soften.

Add the minced ginger and garlic to the skillet and stir-fry for another minute until fragrant.

Stir in the chickpeas, low-sodium soy sauce, and hoisin sauce. Cook for an additional 2 minutes until everything is well combined and heated through.

Serve the chickpea and vegetable stir-fry over cooked brown rice or quinoa, if desired. Garnish with sliced green onions.

Turkey and Avocado Wrap:

Ingredients

4 whole-grain tortillas or wraps

8 slices of lean turkey breast

1 avocado, sliced

1 cup lettuce or spinach leaves

1 medium tomato, sliced

Mustard or low-fat mayo (optional, for added flavor)

Instructions

Lay out the whole-grain tortillas on a clean surface.

Place 2 slices of lean turkey breast on each tortilla, leaving space near the edges.

Layer the avocado slices, lettuce or spinach leaves, and tomato slices on top of the turkey.

If desired, spread a small amount of mustard or low-fat mayo over the fillings.

Tightly roll up the tortillas, tucking in the sides as you go.

Cut each wrap in half diagonally and serve.

Ratatouille:

Ingredients

1 eggplant, diced

1 zucchini, diced

1 yellow squash, diced

1 red bell pepper, diced

1 yellow bell pepper, diced

1 onion, chopped

2 cloves garlic, minced

1 (14.5-ounce) can diced tomatoes, with juices

2 tablespoons tomato paste

1 tablespoon olive oil

1 teaspoon dried thyme

1 teaspoon dried oregano

Salt and pepper to taste

Fresh basil for garnish (optional)

Instructions

In a large pot or Dutch oven, heat the olive oil over medium heat.

Add the chopped onion and garlic. Sauté for about 2 minutes until they become fragrant.

Add the diced eggplant, zucchini, yellow squash, red bell pepper, and yellow bell pepper to the pot.

Stir in the dried thyme, dried oregano, salt, and pepper.

Cook the vegetables for about 5 minutes until they start to soften.

Add the diced tomatoes with their juices and tomato paste to the pot. Stir well to combine.

Reduce the heat to low, cover the pot, and simmer for about 20-25 minutes or until the vegetables are tender.

Stir the ratatouille occasionally to prevent sticking.

Serve the ratatouille hot, and garnish with fresh basil if desired.

Grilled Shrimp and Vegetable Skewers:

Ingredients

1 lb (450g) large shrimp, peeled and deveined

2 bell peppers (red, yellow, or orange), cut into chunks

1 zucchini, sliced into rounds

1 red onion, cut into chunks

2 tablespoons olive oil

2 cloves garlic, minced

1 teaspoon smoked paprika

1/2 teaspoon cayenne pepper (optional)

Salt and pepper to taste

Wooden skewers, soaked in water for 30 minutes

Instructions

Preheat the grill to medium-high heat.

In a bowl, combine the olive oil, minced garlic, smoked paprika, cayenne pepper (if using), salt, and pepper.

Add the shrimp, bell peppers, zucchini, and red onion to the bowl and toss to coat evenly.

Thread the shrimp and vegetables onto the soaked wooden skewers, alternating between shrimp and vegetables.

Grill the skewers for about 2-3 minutes per side or until the shrimp are cooked through and the vegetables are slightly charred.

Remove from the grill and serve the grilled shrimp and vegetable skewers hot.

Roasted Chicken Breast with Steamed Broccoli:

Ingredients

2 boneless, skinless chicken breasts

2 cups broccoli florets

2 tablespoons olive oil

2 cloves garlic, minced

1 teaspoon dried herbs (such as rosemary, thyme, or oregano)

Salt and pepper to taste

Instructions

Preheat the oven to 400°F (200°C).

Place the chicken breasts on a baking sheet lined with parchment paper.

In a small bowl, mix together the olive oil, minced garlic, dried herbs, salt, and pepper.

Brush the seasoned oil mixture onto both sides of the chicken breasts.

Roast the chicken in the preheated oven for about 20-25 minutes or until cooked through and no longer pink in the center.

While the chicken is roasting, steam the broccoli florets until tender-crisp.

Serve the roasted chicken breast with steamed broccoli on the side.

Tofu and Vegetable Stir-Fry:

Ingredients

1 block firm tofu, pressed and cubed

2 tablespoons low-sodium soy sauce

1 tablespoon cornstarch

1 tablespoon vegetable oil

2 cloves garlic, minced

1 teaspoon grated ginger

2 cups mixed vegetables (such as bell peppers, snow peas, and carrots), sliced

2 green onions, sliced

1 tablespoon hoisin sauce (optional)

Salt and pepper to taste

Instructions

In a bowl, combine the cubed tofu, low-sodium soy sauce, and cornstarch. Toss gently to coat the tofu.

Heat the vegetable oil in a large skillet or wok over medium-high heat.

Add the minced garlic and grated ginger to the skillet and sauté until fragrant.

Add the tofu to the skillet and cook until lightly browned and crispy.

Push the tofu to one side of the skillet and add the mixed vegetables to the other side. Stir-fry for about 5-7 minutes or until the vegetables are tender-crisp.

Stir in the sliced green onions and hoisin sauce (if using). Season with salt and pepper.

Cook for another 2-3 minutes to combine the flavors.

Remove from heat and serve the tofu and vegetable stir-fry hot.

Black Bean and Corn Salad:

Ingredients

1 can black beans, drained and rinsed

1 cup corn kernels (fresh or frozen)

1 bell pepper (red, yellow, or orange), diced

1/2 red onion, finely chopped

1 jalapeño pepper, seeded and minced

2 tablespoons fresh lime juice

2 tablespoons extra-virgin olive oil

1 tablespoon chopped fresh cilantro

Salt and pepper to taste

Instructions

In a large bowl, combine the black beans, corn kernels, diced bell pepper, finely chopped red onion, and minced jalapeño pepper.

In a small bowl, whisk together the fresh lime juice, extra-virgin olive oil, chopped fresh cilantro, salt, and pepper.

Pour the dressing over the black bean mixture and toss to combine.

Adjust the seasoning if needed.

Let the black bean and corn salad sit for a few minutes before serving. Serve chilled.

Grilled Portobello Mushroom Burger with Lettuce Wrap:

Ingredients

4 large Portobello mushroom caps

2 tablespoons balsamic vinegar

2 tablespoons olive oil

2 cloves garlic, minced

Salt and pepper to taste

4 large lettuce leaves (such as butter lettuce or romaine)

Sliced tomatoes, onions, and avocado for topping (optional)

Instructions

Preheat the grill to medium-high heat.

In a small bowl, whisk together the balsamic vinegar, olive oil, minced garlic, salt, and pepper.

Brush both sides of the Portobello mushroom caps with the marinade.

Grill the mushroom caps for about 4-5 minutes per side or until tender and grill marks appear.

Remove the mushroom caps from the grill and let them cool slightly.

Place each grilled Portobello mushroom cap on a lettuce leaf and top with sliced tomatoes, onions, and avocado if desired.

Wrap the lettuce around the mushroom cap to serve the grilled Portobello mushroom burger.

Lemon Herb Roasted Turkey Breast with Roasted Sweet Potatoes:

Ingredients

1 lb (450g) turkey breast, boneless and skinless

2 tablespoons fresh lemon juice

2 tablespoons olive oil

2 cloves garlic, minced

1 teaspoon dried herbs (such as rosemary, thyme, or sage)

Salt and pepper to taste

2 medium sweet potatoes, peeled and cubed

1 tablespoon melted coconut oil

1/2 teaspoon smoked paprika

1/2 teaspoon garlic powder

Salt and pepper to taste

Instructions

Preheat the oven to 375°F (190°C).

In a small bowl, whisk together the fresh lemon juice, olive oil, minced garlic, dried herbs, salt, and pepper.

Place the turkey breast in a baking dish and pour the lemon herb mixture over it. Make sure the turkey breast is evenly coated.

Roast the turkey breast in the preheated oven for about 25-30 minutes or until cooked through and no longer pink in the center.

While the turkey is roasting, toss the cubed sweet potatoes with melted coconut oil, smoked paprika, garlic powder, salt, and pepper in a separate baking dish.

Roast the sweet potatoes for about 20-25 minutes or until tender and lightly browned.

Remove the turkey breast and sweet potatoes from the oven. Let them cool slightly before serving.

Spinach and Feta Stuffed Chicken Breast:

Ingredients

2 boneless, skinless chicken breasts

2 cups fresh spinach leaves

1/4 cup crumbled feta cheese

2 cloves garlic, minced

1 tablespoon olive oil

Salt and pepper to taste

Instructions

Preheat the oven to 400°F (200°C).

Slice each chicken breast horizontally to create a pocket for the filling. Be careful not to cut all the way through.

In a skillet, heat the olive oil over medium heat.

Add the minced garlic and sauté until fragrant.

Add the fresh spinach leaves to the skillet and cook until wilted.

Remove the skillet from heat and stir in the crumbled feta cheese. Season with salt and pepper.

Stuff each chicken breast with the spinach and feta mixture, then secure with toothpicks if needed.

Place the stuffed chicken breasts on a baking sheet lined with parchment paper.

Bake for about 20-25 minutes or until the chicken is cooked through and no longer pink in the center.

Remove the toothpicks before serving the spinach and feta stuffed chicken breast.

Cauliflower Fried Rice with Shrimp:

Ingredients

1 medium head cauliflower, grated or processed into rice-like texture

1 lb (450g) shrimp, peeled and deveined

2 tablespoons low-sodium soy sauce

1 tablespoon sesame oil

1 tablespoon vegetable oil

1 cup mixed vegetables (such as peas, carrots, and bell peppers), diced

2 cloves garlic, minced

2 green onions, sliced

2 eggs, beaten

Salt and pepper to taste

Instructions

In a bowl, marinate the shrimp with low-sodium soy sauce, sesame oil, salt, and pepper. Set aside for about 10 minutes.

Heat the vegetable oil in a large skillet or wok over medium-high heat.

Add the marinated shrimp to the skillet and cook until pink and cooked through. Remove from the skillet and set aside.

In the same skillet, add the minced garlic and diced mixed vegetables. Stir-fry for about 3-4 minutes until the vegetables are tender-crisp.

Push the vegetables to one side of the skillet and add the beaten eggs to the other side. Scramble the eggs until cooked through.

Add the grated cauliflower rice to the skillet and stir-fry for about 3-4 minutes or until heated through.

Stir in the cooked shrimp and sliced green onions. Season with salt and pepper.

Cook for another 1-2 minutes to combine the flavors.

Remove from heat and serve the cauliflower fried rice with shrimp hot.

Greek Yogurt Chicken Salad Lettuce Wraps:

Ingredients

2 cups cooked chicken breast, shredded

1/2 cup Greek yogurt

1/4 cup diced celery

1/4 cup diced red onion

1/4 cup chopped fresh dill

2 tablespoons lemon juice

Salt and pepper to taste

Large lettuce leaves for wrapping

Instructions

In a bowl, combine the shredded chicken breast, Greek yogurt, diced celery, diced red onion, chopped fresh dill, lemon juice, salt, and pepper.

Stir well to thoroughly coat the chicken with the yogurt mixture.

Adjust the seasoning if needed.

Spoon the Greek yogurt chicken salad onto large lettuce leaves.

Wrap the lettuce around the chicken salad filling. Serve the Greek yogurt chicken salad lettuce wraps.

Vegetable and Lentil Curry:

Ingredients

1 cup dried lentils, rinsed

1 tablespoon vegetable oil

1 onion, chopped

2 cloves garlic, minced

1 tablespoon grated ginger

1 tablespoon curry powder

1 teaspoon ground cumin

1 teaspoon ground coriander

1 can (14 oz/400g) diced tomatoes

1 can (14 oz/400g) coconut milk

2 cups mixed vegetables (such as cauliflower, bell peppers, and peas), diced

Salt and pepper to taste

Fresh cilantro leaves for garnish (optional)

Cooked brown rice or whole wheat naan for serving

Instructions

In a large pot, cook the lentils according to the package instructions until tender. Drain and set aside.

In the same pot, heat the vegetable oil over medium heat.

Add the chopped onion, minced garlic, and grated ginger to the pot. Sauté until fragrant.

Stir in the curry powder, ground cumin, and ground coriander. Cook for another minute to toast the spices.

Add the diced tomatoes and coconut milk to the pot. Stir to combine.

Bring the mixture to a boil, then reduce the heat and let it simmer for about 10 minutes to allow the flavors to meld.

Add the cooked lentils and mixed vegetables to the pot. Season with salt and pepper.

Simmer for an additional 10-15 minutes or until the vegetables are tender.

Garnish with fresh cilantro leaves if desired.

Serve the vegetable and lentil curry with cooked brown rice or whole wheat naan.

Quinoa and Black Bean Salad:

Ingredients

1 cup cooked quinoa

1 can (15 oz/425g) black beans, drained and rinsed

1 cup cherry tomatoes, halved

1/2 cup diced red bell pepper

1/4 cup diced red onion

1/4 cup chopped fresh cilantro

2 tablespoons fresh lime juice

2 tablespoons extra-virgin olive oil

1 teaspoon ground cumin

Salt and pepper to taste

Instructions

In a large bowl, combine the cooked quinoa, black beans, cherry tomatoes, diced red bell pepper, diced red onion, and chopped fresh cilantro.

In a small bowl, whisk together the fresh lime juice, extra-virgin olive oil, ground cumin, salt, and pepper.

Pour the dressing over the quinoa and black bean mixture. Toss to coat evenly.

Adjust the seasoning if needed.

Let the quinoa and black bean salad sit for a few minutes to allow the flavors to meld. Serve chilled.

Grilled Tuna Steak with Tomato and Cucumber Salad:

Ingredients

2 tuna steaks

1 tablespoon olive oil

1 teaspoon dried herbs (such as thyme, rosemary, or oregano)

Salt and pepper to taste

1 cup cherry tomatoes, halved

1 cucumber, diced

1/4 red onion, thinly sliced

2 tablespoons fresh lemon juice

2 tablespoons extra-virgin olive oil

1 tablespoon chopped fresh parsley

Salt and pepper to taste

Instructions

Preheat the grill to medium-high heat.

Brush the tuna steaks with olive oil, then sprinkle with dried herbs, salt, and pepper.

Grill the tuna steaks for about 2-3 minutes per side for medium-rare doneness, or adjust the cooking time according to your preference.

Remove the tuna steaks from the grill and let them rest for a few minutes.

In a bowl, combine the cherry tomatoes, diced cucumber, thinly sliced red onion, fresh lemon juice, extra-virgin olive oil, chopped fresh parsley, salt, and pepper.

Toss the ingredients to combine and coat evenly.

Slice the grilled tuna steaks and serve them with the tomato and cucumber salad.

Roasted Vegetable Wrap with Hummus:

Ingredients

2 large whole wheat tortillas

2 cups mixed roasted vegetables (such as eggplant, zucchini, bell peppers, and onions), sliced

1/4 cup hummus

1/4 cup crumbled feta cheese

Fresh spinach leaves

Salt and pepper to taste

Instructions

Lay out the whole wheat tortillas and spread hummus evenly on each tortilla.

Arrange the mixed roasted vegetables on top of the hummus.

Sprinkle crumbled feta cheese over the vegetables.

Place fresh spinach leaves on top.

Season with salt and pepper.

Roll up the tortillas tightly and cut them in half. Serve the roasted vegetable wraps.

Zucchini Noodles with Tomato and Basil Sauce:

Ingredients

2 large zucchini

2 tablespoons olive oil

2 cloves garlic, minced

1 can (14 oz/400g) diced tomatoes

1/4 cup chopped fresh basil leaves

Salt and pepper to taste

Grated Parmesan cheese for topping (optional)

Instructions

Trim the ends of the zucchini, then use a spiralizer or a julienne peeler to create zucchini noodles.

Heat the olive oil in a large skillet over medium heat.

Add the minced garlic to the skillet and sauté until fragrant.

Add the zucchini noodles to the skillet and cook for about 2-3 minutes until tender but still slightly crisp.

Stir in the diced tomatoes and chopped fresh basil.

Season with salt and pepper.

Cook for another 2-3 minutes to heat through.

Remove from heat and serve the zucchini noodles with tomato and basil sauce.

Top with grated Parmesan cheese if desired.

Steamed Fish with Steamed Asparagus:

Ingredients

2 white fish fillets (such as cod, tilapia, or sole)

1 lemon, sliced

Salt and pepper to taste

1 bunch asparagus, trimmed

1 tablespoon olive oil

Lemon wedges for serving

Instructions

Place the fish fillets on a plate and season them with salt and pepper.

Lay the lemon slices on top of the fish fillets.

Prepare a steamer or a steaming basket and bring the water to a simmer.

Place the fish fillets on the steamer rack and cover.

Steam the fish for about 8-10 minutes or until cooked through and flaky.

While the fish is steaming, place the trimmed asparagus in another steamer rack and steam for about 5-7 minutes or until tender-crisp.

Remove the fish and asparagus from the steamer.

Drizzle the steamed asparagus with olive oil and season with salt and pepper.

Serve the steamed fish with steamed asparagus and lemon wedges.

DINNER RECIPES YOU SHOULD TRY!

Baked Salmon with Roasted Vegetables:

Ingredients

4 salmon fillets

2 cups of mixed vegetables (e.g., carrots, bell peppers, zucchini)

2 tablespoons olive oil

1 teaspoon dried thyme

1 teaspoon dried rosemary

Salt and pepper to taste

Instructions

Preheat the oven to 400°F (200°C).

Toss the mixed vegetables with 1 tablespoon of olive oil, dried thyme, dried rosemary, salt, and pepper.

Place the seasoned vegetables on a baking sheet and bake for 15 minutes.

Rub the salmon fillets with the remaining olive oil, salt, and pepper.

After 15 minutes, add the salmon fillets to the baking sheet with the vegetables.

Bake for an additional 10-12 minutes or until the salmon is cooked through.

Grilled Chicken Breast with Quinoa and Steamed Broccoli:

Ingredients

4 boneless, skinless chicken breasts

1 cup quinoa

2 cups water or low-sodium chicken broth

2 cups broccoli florets

2 tablespoons olive oil

1 teaspoon garlic powder

Salt and pepper to taste

Instructions

Preheat the grill to medium-high heat.

Season the chicken breasts with olive oil, garlic powder, salt, and pepper.

Grill the chicken for 6-8 minutes per side or until cooked through.

While the chicken is grilling, rinse the quinoa under cold water and cook it in water or chicken broth according to package instructions.

Steam the broccoli until tender, about 5-7 minutes.

Serve the grilled chicken over a bed of cooked quinoa with steamed broccoli on the side.

Lentil Soup with Whole-Grain Bread:

Ingredients

1 cup dried green lentils

1 onion, chopped

2 carrots, diced

2 celery stalks, diced

2 cloves garlic, minced

6 cups low-sodium vegetable broth or water

1 bay leaf

1 teaspoon dried thyme

Salt and pepper to taste

Fresh parsley for garnish (optional)

Instructions

In a large pot, sauté the chopped onion, carrots, and celery in a little olive oil until softened.

Add the minced garlic and cook for another minute.

Rinse the lentils and add them to the pot along with the vegetable broth or water, bay leaf, dried thyme, salt, and pepper.

Bring the soup to a boil, then reduce the heat and simmer for about 25-30 minutes or until the lentils are tender.

Remove the bay leaf before serving.

Garnish with fresh parsley if desired.

Serve the lentil soup with slices of whole-grain bread.

Turkey Chili with a Side Salad:

Ingredients

1 lb ground turkey

1 onion, chopped

1 red bell pepper, chopped

1 can (15 oz) diced tomatoes

1 can (15 oz) kidney beans, drained and rinsed

2 cups low-sodium vegetable broth or water

2 tablespoons chili powder

1 teaspoon cumin

1 teaspoon paprika

Salt and pepper to taste

Mixed salad greens

Cherry tomatoes

Cucumber slices

Balsamic vinaigrette dressing

Instructions

In a large pot, cook the ground turkey until browned.

Add the chopped onion and red bell pepper, and cook until softened.

Stir in the diced tomatoes, kidney beans, vegetable broth or water, chili powder, cumin, paprika, salt, and pepper.

Bring the chili to a boil, then reduce the heat and simmer for about 20-25 minutes.

While the chili is simmering, prepare the side salad by combining mixed salad greens, cherry tomatoes, and cucumber slices.

Drizzle with balsamic vinaigrette dressing.

Serve the turkey chili with the side salad.

Vegetable Stir-Fry with Tofu and Brown Rice:

Ingredients

1 block of firm tofu, cubed

2 cups mixed stir-fry vegetables (e.g., broccoli, bell peppers, snap peas)

2 tablespoons low-sodium soy sauce

1 tablespoon sesame oil

1 tablespoon cornstarch

2 cups cooked brown rice

Instructions

In a bowl, combine the cubed tofu with soy sauce and cornstarch. Let it marinate for a few minutes.

Heat sesame oil in a wok or large skillet over medium-high heat.

Add the marinated tofu and stir-fry until it becomes lightly browned and slightly crispy.

Add the mixed vegetables to the pan and continue to stir-fry until they are tender-crisp.

Serve the tofu and vegetables over cooked brown rice.

Grilled Shrimp with Asparagus and Couscous:

Ingredients

1 lb large shrimp, peeled and deveined

1 bunch of asparagus, trimmed

2 tablespoons olive oil

1 teaspoon lemon zest

1 teaspoon paprika

Salt and pepper to taste

1 cup couscous, cooked according to package instructions

Instructions

Preheat the grill to medium-high heat.

In a bowl, toss the shrimp and asparagus with olive oil, lemon zest, paprika, salt, and pepper.

Grill the shrimp and asparagus for about 2-3 minutes per side until the shrimp are pink and cooked through.

Serve the grilled shrimp and asparagus over a bed of cooked couscous.

Stuffed Bell Peppers with Lean Ground Turkey and Tomatoes:

Ingredients

4 bell peppers (any color)

1 lb lean ground turkey

1 cup cooked quinoa

1 can (15 oz) diced tomatoes

1 teaspoon dried oregano

1 teaspoon dried basil

Salt and pepper to taste

1/2 cup shredded mozzarella cheese (optional)

Instructions

Preheat the oven to 375°F (190°C).

Cut the tops off the bell peppers and remove the seeds and membranes.

In a skillet, cook the ground turkey until browned.

Stir in the cooked quinoa, diced tomatoes, dried oregano, dried basil, salt, and pepper.

Stuff each bell pepper with the turkey and quinoa mixture.

If desired, sprinkle shredded mozzarella cheese on top of each stuffed pepper.

Place the stuffed peppers in a baking dish and bake for about 25-30 minutes or until the peppers are tender.

Baked Cod with Sweet Potato Mash:

Ingredients

4 cod fillets

2 large sweet potatoes, peeled and diced

2 tablespoons olive oil

1/4 cup low-fat milk or almond milk

1 tablespoon unsalted butter (optional)

1 teaspoon garlic powder

Salt and pepper to taste

Instructions

Preheat the oven to 400°F (200°C).

Place the cod fillets on a baking sheet and drizzle with olive oil, garlic powder, salt, and pepper.

Bake the cod for 12-15 minutes or until it flakes easily with a fork.

While the cod is baking, boil the diced sweet potatoes until they are tender.

Drain the sweet potatoes and mash them with milk, butter (if using), salt, and pepper until smooth.

Serve the baked cod with a side of sweet potato mash.

Chickpea and Spinach Curry served with Brown Rice:

Ingredients

1 can (15 oz) chickpeas, drained and rinsed

2 cups fresh spinach leaves

1 onion, chopped

2 cloves garlic, minced

1 can (15 oz) diced tomatoes

1 can (14 oz) coconut milk

1 tablespoon curry powder

1 teaspoon ground cumin

1 teaspoon ground coriander

1 tablespoon vegetable oil

Salt and pepper to taste

Cooked brown rice for serving

Instructions

In a large skillet, heat vegetable oil over medium heat.

Add the chopped onion and garlic, and sauté until softened.

Stir in the curry powder, ground cumin, and ground coriander, and cook for another minute.

Add the chickpeas, diced tomatoes, and coconut milk to the skillet.

Simmer the mixture for about 10 minutes, allowing the flavors to blend.

Add the fresh spinach leaves to the skillet and cook until wilted.

Season the curry with salt and pepper to taste.

Serve the chickpea and spinach curry over cooked brown rice.

Grilled Chicken or Vegetable Skewers with a Side of Mixed Greens:

Ingredients

1 lb boneless, skinless chicken breasts (cut into cubes) OR mixed vegetables (e.g., bell peppers, cherry tomatoes, zucchini, mushrooms)

Wooden or metal skewers

2 tablespoons olive oil

1 tablespoon lemon juice

1 teaspoon dried oregano

Salt and pepper to taste

Mixed salad greens

Balsamic vinaigrette dressing

Instructions

If using wooden skewers, soak them in water for 30 minutes before grilling to prevent burning.

Thread the chicken cubes or vegetables onto the skewers.

In a bowl, whisk together olive oil, lemon juice, dried oregano, salt, and pepper.

Brush the skewers with the olive oil mixture.

Grill the skewers over medium-high heat for about 10-12 minutes, turning occasionally until the chicken is cooked through or the vegetables are tender.

Serve the grilled skewers with a side of mixed salad greens drizzled with balsamic vinaigrette dressing.

Baked Tilapia with Lemon and Dill, accompanied by Roasted Brussels Sprouts:

Ingredients

4 tilapia fillets

1 lemon, sliced

Fresh dill sprigs

2 tablespoons olive oil

Salt and pepper to taste

1 lb Brussels sprouts, trimmed and halved

1 tablespoon balsamic vinegar

Instructions

Preheat the oven to 375°F (190°C).

Place the tilapia fillets on a baking sheet and season with salt and pepper.

Lay lemon slices and dill sprigs on top of each fillet.

Drizzle olive oil over the fish and bake for about 12-15 minutes or until the tilapia is cooked through.

While the tilapia is baking, toss the halved Brussels sprouts with olive oil, salt, and pepper.

Spread the Brussels sprouts on a separate baking sheet and roast in the oven for 15-20 minutes or until they are tender and slightly crispy.

Drizzle balsamic vinegar over the roasted Brussels sprouts before serving.

Zucchini Noodles with a Lean Turkey Bolognese Sauce:

Ingredients

4 large zucchinis, spiralized into noodles

1 lb lean ground turkey

1 onion, chopped

2 cloves garlic, minced

1 can (28 oz) crushed tomatoes

1 teaspoon dried oregano

1 teaspoon dried basil

Salt and pepper to taste

Grated Parmesan cheese for garnish (optional)

Instructions

In a large skillet, cook the ground turkey until browned.

Add the chopped onion and minced garlic, and cook until softened.

Stir in the crushed tomatoes, dried oregano, dried basil, salt, and pepper.

Simmer the Bolognese sauce for about 15-20 minutes, allowing the flavors to meld.

In a separate pan, sauté the zucchini noodles for 2-3 minutes until they are just tender.

Serve the Bolognese sauce over the zucchini noodles and garnish with grated Parmesan cheese if desired.

Spinach and Feta Stuffed Chicken Breast with a Side of Quinoa:

Ingredients

4 boneless, skinless chicken breasts

2 cups fresh spinach leaves

1/2 cup crumbled feta cheese

1 tablespoon olive oil

Salt and pepper to taste

1 cup quinoa, cooked according to package instructions

Instructions

Preheat the oven to 375°F (190°C).

Carefully slice a pocket into each chicken breast.

In a bowl, mix the fresh spinach leaves and crumbled feta cheese.

Stuff each chicken breast with the spinach and feta mixture and secure with toothpicks if needed.

Heat olive oil in an oven-safe skillet over medium-high heat.

Season the stuffed chicken breasts with salt and pepper and sear them for 2-3 minutes on each side.

Transfer the skillet to the preheated oven and bake for about 15-20 minutes or until the chicken is cooked through.

Serve the stuffed chicken breasts with a side of cooked quinoa.

Eggplant and Tomato Gratin with a Sprinkle of Parmesan Cheese:

Ingredients

1 large eggplant, sliced into rounds

2 large tomatoes, sliced

2 cloves garlic, minced

1 tablespoon olive oil

1 teaspoon dried thyme

Salt and pepper to taste

1/4 cup grated Parmesan cheese

Instructions

Preheat the oven to 375°F (190°C).

In a baking dish, layer the sliced eggplant and tomatoes.

Sprinkle minced garlic, dried thyme, salt, and pepper over the vegetables.

Drizzle olive oil over the top.

Cover the baking dish with foil and bake for about 20 minutes.

Remove the foil, sprinkle grated Parmesan cheese on top, and bake for an additional 10-15 minutes or until the cheese is melted and slightly golden.

Tofu and Vegetable Kebabs served with a Cucumber-Tomato Salad:

Ingredients

1 block of firm tofu, cut into cubes

Assorted vegetables (e.g., bell peppers, cherry tomatoes, red onions, zucchini), cut into chunks

Wooden or metal skewers

2 tablespoons olive oil

1 tablespoon balsamic vinegar

1 teaspoon dried oregano

Salt and pepper to taste

1 cucumber, diced

1 cup cherry tomatoes, halved

1/4 cup red onion, thinly sliced

2 tablespoons fresh lemon juice

Fresh parsley for garnish (optional)

Instructions

If using wooden skewers, soak them in water for 30 minutes before grilling to prevent burning.

Thread the tofu cubes and vegetable chunks onto the skewers.

In a bowl, whisk together olive oil, balsamic vinegar, dried oregano, salt, and pepper.

Brush the kebabs with the olive oil mixture.

Grill the kebabs over medium-high heat for about 8-10 minutes, turning occasionally until the tofu is lightly browned and the vegetables are tender.

In a separate bowl, combine the diced cucumber, cherry tomatoes, and sliced red onion.

Drizzle fresh lemon juice over the salad and toss to combine.

Garnish the salad with fresh parsley if desired.

Serve the tofu and vegetable kebabs with the cucumber-tomato salad.

Black Bean and Sweet Potato Enchiladas with a Side of Guacamole:

Ingredients

8 whole wheat tortillas

1 can (15 oz) black beans, drained and rinsed

2 cups cooked and mashed sweet potatoes

1 cup diced bell peppers (any color)

1 cup diced onions

2 cloves garlic, minced

1 tablespoon olive oil

1 teaspoon ground cumin

1 teaspoon chili powder

Salt and pepper to taste

1 cup enchilada sauce (store-bought or homemade)

1 cup shredded cheddar or Mexican blend cheese

Guacamole for serving

Instructions

Preheat the oven to 375°F (190°C).

In a skillet, heat olive oil over medium heat.

Add diced onions, garlic, and diced bell peppers, and cook until softened.

Stir in black beans, mashed sweet potatoes, ground cumin, chili powder, salt, and pepper. Cook until well combined and heated through.

Spoon the mixture onto each whole wheat tortilla and roll it up, placing it seam-side down in a baking dish.

Pour enchilada sauce over the rolled tortillas and sprinkle shredded cheese on top.

Cover the baking dish with foil and bake for about 15-20 minutes, removing the foil for the last 5 minutes to brown the cheese.

Serve the black bean and sweet potato enchiladas with a side of guacamole.

Poached Chicken with a Lemon-Herb Sauce and Steamed Green Beans:

Ingredients

4 boneless, skinless chicken breasts

2 cups low-sodium chicken broth or water

1 lemon, juiced and zested

2 tablespoons chopped fresh herbs (e.g., parsley, thyme, rosemary)

1 tablespoon olive oil

Salt and pepper to taste

1 lb fresh green beans

Instructions

In a large saucepan, bring the chicken broth or water to a simmer.

Add the chicken breasts to the simmering liquid and poach them for about 12-15 minutes or until cooked through.

In a small bowl, whisk together lemon juice, lemon zest, chopped herbs, olive oil, salt, and pepper to make the lemon-herb sauce.

Steam the green beans until they are tender-crisp.

Serve the poached chicken with a drizzle of the lemon-herb sauce and a side of steamed green beans.

Cauliflower Rice Stir-Fry with Shrimp or Tofu and a Medley of Veggies:

Ingredients

1 head cauliflower, grated or processed into "rice"

1 lb shrimp, peeled and deveined OR tofu, cubed

2 cups mixed stir-fry vegetables (e.g., broccoli, bell peppers, snap peas, carrots)

2 tablespoons low-sodium soy sauce

1 tablespoon sesame oil

1 tablespoon hoisin sauce (optional)

2 cloves garlic, minced

1 tablespoon vegetable oil

Salt and pepper to taste

Instructions

In a large skillet or wok, heat vegetable oil over medium-high heat.

If using shrimp, stir-fry them until pink and cooked through. If using tofu, stir-fry until lightly browned.

Add the mixed stir-fry vegetables and minced garlic to the skillet and stir-fry until the vegetables are tender-crisp.

Push the shrimp or tofu and vegetables to one side of the skillet and add the cauliflower rice to the other side.

Drizzle sesame oil, soy sauce, and hoisin sauce (if using) over the cauliflower rice, and stir-fry it until heated through and slightly softened.

Mix the cauliflower rice with the shrimp or tofu and vegetables in the skillet.

Season with salt and pepper to taste.

Serve the cauliflower rice stir-fry with shrimp or tofu and a medley of veggies.

Baked Chicken and Vegetable Foil Packets Seasoned with Herbs:

Ingredients

4 boneless, skinless chicken breasts

2 cups chopped mixed vegetables (e.g., bell peppers, zucchini, cherry tomatoes)

2 tablespoons olive oil

1 teaspoon dried thyme

1 teaspoon dried rosemary

1 teaspoon garlic powder

Salt and pepper to taste

Instructions

Preheat the oven to 400°F (200°C).

Cut four pieces of aluminum foil, large enough to wrap around each chicken breast and vegetables.

In a bowl, toss the chopped vegetables with olive oil, dried thyme, dried rosemary, garlic powder, salt, and pepper.

Place each chicken breast on a piece of foil and surround it with the seasoned vegetables.

Fold and seal each foil packet, leaving some space inside for steam.

Place the foil packets on a baking sheet and bake for about 20-25 minutes or until the chicken is cooked through and the vegetables are tender.

Quinoa and Kale Salad with Grilled Chicken and a Light Vinaigrette Dressing:

Ingredients

4 boneless, skinless chicken breasts

1 cup quinoa, cooked according to package instructions

2 cups chopped kale leaves

1 cup cherry tomatoes, halved

1/2 cup chopped cucumber

1/4 cup chopped red onion

2 tablespoons chopped fresh parsley

2 tablespoons olive oil

2 tablespoons balsamic vinegar

1 teaspoon Dijon mustard

Salt and pepper to taste

Instructions

Preheat the grill to medium-high heat.

Season the chicken breasts with olive oil, salt, and pepper.

Grill the chicken for 6-8 minutes per side or until cooked through.

In a large bowl, combine the cooked quinoa, chopped kale, cherry tomatoes, cucumber, red onion, and chopped parsley.

In a separate small bowl, whisk together olive oil, balsamic vinegar, Dijon mustard, salt, and pepper to make the vinaigrette dressing.

Pour the dressing over the quinoa and kale salad, tossing to coat the ingredients.

Slice the grilled chicken and serve it on top of the quinoa and kale salad.

SOUP RECIPES YOU SHOULD TRY!

Minestrone Soup:

Ingredients

1 tablespoon olive oil

1 medium onion, chopped

2 garlic cloves, minced

2 medium carrots, diced

2 celery stalks, diced

1 medium zucchini, diced

1 cup chopped green beans

1 can (14 oz) diced tomatoes (low-sodium)

4 cups low-sodium vegetable broth

1 can (15 oz) kidney beans, drained and rinsed

1 teaspoon dried oregano

1 teaspoon dried basil

Salt and pepper to taste

1 cup cooked whole wheat pasta (e.g., macaroni, penne, or shells)

Grated Parmesan cheese for garnish (optional)

Instructions

In a large pot, heat the olive oil over medium heat. Add the chopped onions and garlic, sauté until fragrant.

Add the diced carrots, celery, zucchini, and green beans. Cook for a few minutes until slightly softened.

Stir in the diced tomatoes, vegetable broth, kidney beans, dried oregano, and dried basil.

Bring the soup to a boil, then reduce the heat to low and let it simmer for about 15-20 minutes.

Season with salt and pepper to taste. Add the cooked pasta to the soup.

Serve hot, and if desired, garnish with grated Parmesan cheese.

Tomato Basil Soup (with low-sodium broth):

Ingredients

1 tablespoon olive oil

1 medium onion, chopped

2 garlic cloves, minced

4 cups low-sodium vegetable broth

2 cans (28 oz each) whole peeled tomatoes (low-sodium), with juice

1/2 cup fresh basil leaves, chopped

1/2 cup low-fat milk or almond milk

Salt and pepper to taste

Fresh basil leaves for garnish

Instructions

In a large pot, heat the olive oil over medium heat. Add the chopped onions and garlic, sauté until fragrant.

Add the vegetable broth and the canned tomatoes (with their juice) to the pot. Break the tomatoes into smaller pieces using a spoon.

Simmer the soup for about 20 minutes, stirring occasionally.

Stir in the chopped basil and let it simmer for another 5 minutes.

Using an immersion blender or a regular blender (in batches), blend the soup until smooth.

Stir in the low-fat milk or almond milk and heat the soup for a few more minutes until warmed through.

Season with salt and pepper to taste. Garnish with fresh basil leaves before serving.

Chicken and Vegetable Soup (using lean chicken breast):

Ingredients

1 tablespoon olive oil

1 pound boneless, skinless chicken breasts, cut into bite-sized pieces

1 medium onion, chopped

2 garlic cloves, minced

2 medium carrots, diced

2 celery stalks, diced

1 medium zucchini, diced

4 cups low-sodium chicken broth

2 cups water

1 teaspoon dried thyme

1 bay leaf

Salt and pepper to taste

Fresh parsley for garnish

Instructions

In a large pot, heat the olive oil over medium heat. Add the chopped onions and garlic, sauté until fragrant.

Add the diced chicken pieces to the pot and cook until browned on all sides.

Stir in the diced carrots, celery, zucchini, chicken broth, water, dried thyme, and bay leaf.

Bring the soup to a boil, then reduce the heat to low and let it simmer for about 20-25 minutes.

Season with salt and pepper to taste. Remove the bay leaf before serving.

Garnish with fresh parsley before serving.

Mushroom Barley Soup:

Ingredients

1 tablespoon olive oil

1 medium onion, chopped

2 garlic cloves, minced

8 oz cremini or button mushrooms, sliced

1/2 cup pearl barley

4 cups low-sodium vegetable broth

2 cups water

2 carrots, diced

2 celery stalks, diced

1 teaspoon dried thyme

Salt and pepper to taste

Fresh parsley for garnish

Instructions

In a large pot, heat the olive oil over medium heat. Add the chopped onions and garlic, sauté until fragrant.

Add the sliced mushrooms to the pot and cook until they release their moisture and turn slightly brown.

Stir in the pearl barley, vegetable broth, water, diced carrots, diced celery, and dried thyme.

Bring the soup to a boil, then reduce the heat to low and let it simmer for about 30-35 minutes or until the barley is tender.

Season with salt and pepper to taste. Garnish with fresh parsley before serving.

Spinach and White Bean Soup:

Ingredients

1 tablespoon olive oil

1 medium onion, chopped

2 garlic cloves, minced

4 cups low-sodium vegetable broth

2 cans (15 oz each) cannellini beans, drained and rinsed

1 bunch fresh spinach leaves, chopped

1 teaspoon dried oregano

1/2 teaspoon crushed red pepper flakes (optional)

Salt and pepper to taste

Grated Parmesan cheese for garnish (optional)

Instructions

In a large pot, heat the olive oil over medium heat. Add the chopped onions and garlic, sauté until fragrant.

Add the vegetable broth and cannellini beans to the pot. Bring to a boil, then reduce the heat to low and let it simmer for about 10-15 minutes.

Stir in the chopped spinach, dried oregano, and crushed red pepper flakes (if using).

Simmer the soup for another 5 minutes until the spinach wilts.

Season with salt and pepper to taste. If desired, garnish with grated Parmesan cheese before serving.

Quinoa and Vegetable Soup:

Ingredients

1 tablespoon olive oil

1 medium onion, chopped

2 garlic cloves, minced

2 medium carrots, diced

2 celery stalks, diced

1 medium zucchini, diced

1/2 cup quinoa, rinsed

4 cups low-sodium vegetable broth

2 cups water

1 teaspoon dried thyme

Salt and pepper to taste

Fresh parsley for garnish

Instructions

In a large pot, heat the olive oil over medium heat. Add the chopped onions and garlic, sauté until fragrant.

Add the diced carrots, celery, zucchini, and rinsed quinoa to the pot.

Stir in the vegetable broth, water, and dried thyme.

Bring the soup to a boil, then reduce the heat to low and let it simmer for about 15-20 minutes or until the quinoa and vegetables are tender.

Season with salt and pepper to taste. Garnish with fresh parsley before serving.

Split Pea Soup (low in sodium):

Ingredients

1 tablespoon olive oil

1 medium onion, chopped

2 garlic cloves, minced

2 cups dried split peas, rinsed

4 cups low-sodium vegetable broth

2 cups water

2 medium carrots, diced

2 celery stalks, diced

1 teaspoon dried thyme

Salt and pepper to taste

Fresh parsley for garnish

Instructions

In a large pot, heat the olive oil over medium heat. Add the chopped onions and garlic, sauté until fragrant.

Add the rinsed split peas, vegetable broth, water, diced carrots, diced celery, and dried thyme to the pot.

Bring the soup to a boil, then reduce the heat to low and let it simmer for about 40-45 minutes or until the split peas are soft.

Season with salt and pepper to taste. Garnish with fresh parsley before serving.

Turkey Chili Soup:

Ingredients

1 tablespoon olive oil

1 medium onion, chopped

2 garlic cloves, minced

1 pound lean ground turkey

1 can (14 oz) diced tomatoes (low-sodium)

1 can (15 oz) kidney beans, drained and rinsed

4 cups low-sodium chicken broth

2 teaspoons chili powder

1 teaspoon ground cumin

Salt and pepper to taste

Fresh cilantro for garnish

Instructions

In a large pot, heat the olive oil over medium heat. Add the chopped onions and garlic, sauté until fragrant.

Add the ground turkey to the pot and cook until browned.

Stir in the diced tomatoes, kidney beans, chicken broth, chili powder, and ground cumin.

Bring the soup to a boil, then reduce the heat to low and let it simmer for about 20-25 minutes.

Season with salt and pepper to taste. Garnish with fresh cilantro before serving.

Butternut Squash Soup (without excessive cream):

Ingredients

1 tablespoon olive oil

1 medium onion, chopped

2 garlic cloves, minced

1 butternut squash, peeled, seeded, and diced

4 cups low-sodium vegetable broth

1 cup water

1/2 teaspoon ground cinnamon

1/4 teaspoon ground nutmeg

Salt and pepper to taste

Roasted pumpkin seeds for garnish (optional)

Instructions

In a large pot, heat the olive oil over medium heat. Add the chopped onions and garlic, sauté until fragrant.

Add the diced butternut squash to the pot and cook for a few minutes until slightly softened.

Stir in the vegetable broth, water, ground cinnamon, and ground nutmeg.

Bring the soup to a boil, then reduce the heat to low and let it simmer for about 20-25 minutes or until the butternut squash is tender.

Using an immersion blender or a regular blender (in batches), blend the soup until smooth.

Season with salt and pepper to taste. If desired, garnish with roasted pumpkin seeds before serving.

Gazpacho (cold tomato-based soup):

Ingredients

6 ripe tomatoes, diced

1 cucumber, peeled and diced

1 red bell pepper, diced

1 small red onion, chopped

2 garlic cloves, minced

2 cups tomato juice (low-sodium)

2 tablespoons red wine vinegar

2 tablespoons olive oil

1 teaspoon ground cumin

Salt and pepper to taste

Fresh basil leaves for garnish

Instructions

In a large bowl, combine the diced tomatoes, cucumber, red bell pepper, chopped red onion, and minced garlic.

Add the tomato juice, red wine vinegar, olive oil, ground cumin, salt, and pepper to the bowl. Stir well to combine.

Using a blender or a food processor, blend half of the mixture until smooth.

Combine the blended mixture with the remaining diced vegetables. Stir well.

Chill the gazpacho in the refrigerator for at least 2 hours before serving.

Garnish with fresh basil leaves before serving.

Cabbage Soup (using lean meats or vegetarian):

Ingredients

1 tablespoon olive oil

1 medium onion, chopped

2 garlic cloves, minced

4 cups low-sodium vegetable or chicken broth

4 cups shredded green cabbage

2 medium carrots, diced

2 celery stalks, diced

1 can (14 oz) diced tomatoes (low-sodium)

1 bay leaf

1 teaspoon dried thyme

Salt and pepper to taste

Fresh parsley for garnish

Instructions

In a large pot, heat the olive oil over medium heat. Add the chopped onions and garlic, sauté until fragrant.

Add the shredded cabbage, diced carrots, diced celery, diced tomatoes (with their juice), vegetable or chicken broth, bay leaf, and dried thyme.

Bring the soup to a boil, then reduce the heat to low and let it simmer for about 15-20 minutes or until the vegetables are tender.

Season with salt and pepper to taste. Remove the bay leaf before serving.

Garnish with fresh parsley before serving.

Black Bean Soup (low in sodium):

Ingredients

1 tablespoon olive oil

1 medium onion, chopped

2 garlic cloves, minced

2 cans (15 oz each) black beans, drained and rinsed (low-sodium)

4 cups low-sodium vegetable or chicken broth

1 can (14 oz) diced tomatoes (low-sodium)

1 teaspoon ground cumin

1/2 teaspoon chili powder

Salt and pepper to taste

Fresh cilantro for garnish

Instructions

In a large pot, heat the olive oil over medium heat. Add the chopped onions and garlic, sauté until fragrant.

Add one can of black beans to the pot and mash them slightly with a fork or a potato masher.

Stir in the second can of whole black beans, vegetable or chicken broth, diced tomatoes (with their juice), ground cumin, and chili powder.

Bring the soup to a boil, then reduce the heat to low and let it simmer for about 10-15 minutes.

Season with salt and pepper to taste. Garnish with fresh cilantro before serving.

Broccoli and Cheese Soup (with reduced-fat cheese):

Ingredients

1 tablespoon olive oil

1 medium onion, chopped

2 garlic cloves, minced

4 cups low-sodium vegetable or chicken broth

4 cups chopped broccoli florets

1 cup shredded reduced-fat cheddar cheese

1/2 cup low-fat milk or almond milk

Salt and pepper to taste

Instructions

In a large pot, heat the olive oil over medium heat. Add the chopped onions and garlic, sauté until fragrant.

Add the chopped broccoli florets and cook for a few minutes until they start to soften.

Stir in the vegetable or chicken broth and bring the soup to a boil.

Reduce the heat to low and let it simmer for about 15-20 minutes or until the broccoli is tender.

Using an immersion blender or a regular blender (in batches), blend the soup until smooth.

Return the blended soup to the pot and stir in the shredded reduced-fat cheddar cheese and low-fat milk or almond milk.

Heat the soup for a few more minutes until the cheese is melted and the soup is warmed through.

Season with salt and pepper to taste.

Chickpea and Vegetable Soup:

Ingredients

1 tablespoon olive oil

1 medium onion, chopped

2 garlic cloves, minced

2 medium carrots, diced

2 celery stalks, diced

1 red bell pepper, diced

1 can (14 oz) diced tomatoes (low-sodium)

1 can (15 oz) chickpeas, drained and rinsed

4 cups low-sodium vegetable broth

2 teaspoons ground cumin

1 teaspoon ground coriander

Salt and pepper to taste

Fresh cilantro for garnish

Instructions

In a large pot, heat the olive oil over medium heat. Add the chopped onions and garlic, sauté until fragrant.

Add the diced carrots, diced celery, and diced red bell pepper to the pot. Cook for a few minutes until they start to soften.

Stir in the diced tomatoes, chickpeas, vegetable broth, ground cumin, and ground coriander.

Bring the soup to a boil, then reduce the heat to low and let it simmer for about 15-20 minutes.

Season with salt and pepper to taste. Garnish with fresh cilantro before serving.

Cauliflower Soup (without excessive cream or butter):

Ingredients

1 tablespoon olive oil

1 medium onion, chopped

2 garlic cloves, minced

1 head cauliflower, chopped into florets

4 cups low-sodium vegetable or chicken broth

2 cups water

1/2 cup low-fat milk or almond milk

Salt and pepper to taste

Fresh chives for garnish

Instructions

In a large pot, heat the olive oil over medium heat. Add the chopped onions and garlic, sauté until fragrant.

Add the chopped cauliflower florets to the pot and cook for a few minutes until they start to soften.

Stir in the vegetable or chicken broth and water.

Bring the soup to a boil, then reduce the heat to low and let it simmer for about 20-25 minutes or until the cauliflower is tender.

Using an immersion blender or a regular blender (in batches), blend the soup until smooth.

Stir in the low-fat milk or almond milk and heat the soup for a few more minutes until warmed through.

Season with salt and pepper to taste. Garnish with fresh chives before serving.

Beetroot and Carrot Soup:

Ingredients

1 tablespoon olive oil

1 medium onion, chopped

2 garlic cloves, minced

3 medium beetroots, peeled and chopped

3 medium carrots, peeled and chopped

4 cups low-sodium vegetable or chicken broth

2 cups water

1 tablespoon balsamic vinegar

Salt and pepper to taste

Greek yogurt or sour cream for garnish (optional)

Instructions

In a large pot, heat the olive oil over medium heat. Add the chopped onions and garlic, sauté until fragrant.

Add the chopped beetroots and chopped carrots to the pot and cook for a few minutes until they start to soften.

Stir in the vegetable or chicken broth and water.

Bring the soup to a boil, then reduce the heat to low and let it simmer for about 20-25 minutes or until the beetroots and carrots are tender.

Using an immersion blender or a regular blender (in batches), blend the soup until smooth.

Stir in the balsamic vinegar and heat the soup for a few more minutes until warmed through.

Season with salt and pepper to taste. If desired, garnish with a dollop of Greek yogurt or sour cream before serving.

Sweet Potato and Ginger Soup:

Ingredients

1 tablespoon olive oil

1 medium onion, chopped

2 garlic cloves, minced

3 medium sweet potatoes, peeled and chopped

1-inch piece fresh ginger, peeled and minced

4 cups low-sodium vegetable or chicken broth

2 cups water

1/2 cup low-fat coconut milk

Salt and pepper to taste

Fresh cilantro for garnish

Instructions

In a large pot, heat the olive oil over medium heat. Add the chopped onions and garlic, sauté until fragrant.

Add the chopped sweet potatoes and minced ginger to the pot and cook for a few minutes until they start to soften.

Stir in the vegetable or chicken broth and water.

Bring the soup to a boil, then reduce the heat to low and let it simmer for about 20-25 minutes or until the sweet potatoes are tender.

Using an immersion blender or a regular blender (in batches), blend the soup until smooth.

Stir in the low-fat coconut milk and heat the soup for a few more minutes until warmed through.

Season with salt and pepper to taste. Garnish with fresh cilantro before serving.

Pumpkin Soup (with low-fat coconut milk):

Ingredients

1 tablespoon olive oil

1 medium onion, chopped

2 garlic cloves, minced

2 cups pumpkin puree (canned or homemade)

4 cups low-sodium vegetable or chicken broth

2 cups water

1/2 cup low-fat coconut milk

1/2 teaspoon ground cinnamon

1/4 teaspoon ground nutmeg

Salt and pepper to taste

Roasted pumpkin seeds for garnish (optional)

Instructions

In a large pot, heat the olive oil over medium heat. Add the chopped onions and garlic, sauté until fragrant.

Add the pumpkin puree to the pot and cook for a few minutes to enhance its flavor.

Stir in the vegetable or chicken broth and water.

Bring the soup to a boil, then reduce the heat to low and let it simmer for about 10-15 minutes.

Stir in the low-fat coconut milk, ground cinnamon, and ground nutmeg.

Heat the soup for a few more minutes until warmed through.

Season with salt and pepper to taste. If desired, garnish with roasted pumpkin seeds before serving.

Asparagus and Green Pea Soup:

Ingredients

1 tablespoon olive oil

1 medium onion, chopped

2 garlic cloves, minced

1 bunch asparagus, trimmed and chopped

2 cups frozen green peas

4 cups low-sodium vegetable or chicken broth

2 cups water

1 tablespoon fresh lemon juice

Salt and pepper to taste

Fresh dill for garnish

Instructions

In a large pot, heat the olive oil over medium heat. Add the chopped onions and garlic, sauté until fragrant.

Add the chopped asparagus to the pot and cook for a few minutes until slightly softened.

Stir in the frozen green peas, vegetable or chicken broth, and water.

Bring the soup to a boil, then reduce the heat to low and let it simmer for about 10-15 minutes.

Using an immersion blender or a regular blender (in batches), blend the soup until smooth.

Stir in the fresh lemon juice and heat the soup for a few more minutes until warmed through.

Season with salt and pepper to taste. Garnish with fresh dill before serving.

Artichoke and Potato Soup:

Ingredients

1 tablespoon olive oil

1 medium onion, chopped

2 garlic cloves, minced

1 can (14 oz) artichoke hearts, drained and chopped

2 medium potatoes, peeled and diced

4 cups low-sodium vegetable or chicken broth

2 cups water

1/2 cup low-fat milk or almond milk

Salt and pepper to taste

Fresh parsley for garnish

Instructions

In a large pot, heat the olive oil over medium heat. Add the chopped onions and garlic, sauté until fragrant.

Add the chopped artichoke hearts and diced potatoes to the pot and cook for a few minutes until they start to soften.

Stir in the vegetable or chicken broth and water.

Bring the soup to a boil, then reduce the heat to low and let it simmer for about 20-25 minutes or until the potatoes are tender.

Using an immersion blender or a regular blender (in batches), blend the soup until smooth.

Stir in the low-fat milk or almond milk and heat the soup for a few more minutes until warmed through.

Season with salt and pepper to taste. Garnish with fresh parsley before serving.

DESSERT RECIPES YOU SHOULD TRY!

Fruit Salad:

Ingredients

Assorted berries (strawberries, blueberries, raspberries)

Melons (watermelon, cantaloupe, honeydew)

Citrus fruits (oranges, mandarins, grapefruits)

Instructions

Wash and cut the fruits into bite-sized pieces.

Mix all the fruits in a large bowl.

Serve immediately or refrigerate for a chilled dessert.

Baked Cinnamon Apple Slices:

Ingredients

Apples (firm variety like Granny Smith or Honeycrisp)

Ground cinnamon

Oats

Honey or maple syrup (optional)

Instructions

Preheat the oven to 375°F (190°C).

Core and slice the apples into thin slices.

Place the apple slices on a baking sheet lined with parchment paper.

Sprinkle ground cinnamon and oats over the apple slices.

Drizzle honey or maple syrup if desired.

Bake for 15-20 minutes or until the apples are tender and slightly caramelized.

Chia Seed Pudding:

Ingredients

Chia seeds

Almond milk (or any plant-based milk)

Fresh fruits (e.g., berries, sliced bananas)

Honey or agave syrup (optional)

Instructions

In a bowl, mix 1/4 cup of chia seeds with 1 cup of almond milk.

Stir well and let it sit for 10 minutes.

Stir again to avoid clumps, cover the bowl, and refrigerate overnight.

In the morning, the chia seeds will have absorbed the milk and become pudding-like.

Serve with fresh fruits and a drizzle of honey or agave syrup if desired.

Greek Yogurt Parfait:

Ingredients

Greek yogurt (plain or flavored)

Granola

Fresh fruits (e.g., berries, sliced peaches)

Honey (optional)

Instructions

In a tall glass or bowl, layer Greek yogurt, granola, and fresh fruits.

Repeat the layers until the glass is filled.

Drizzle honey on top for added sweetness if desired.

Dark Chocolate-Dipped Strawberries:

Ingredients

Fresh strawberries

Dark chocolate chips or chopped dark chocolate

Instructions

Wash and dry the strawberries thoroughly.

Melt the dark chocolate in a microwave-safe bowl or using a double boiler.

Dip each strawberry into the melted chocolate, coating about two-thirds of the fruit.

Place the dipped strawberries on a parchment-lined tray.

Refrigerate until the chocolate hardens.

Baked Pears:

Ingredients

Pears (firm but ripe)

Honey

Ground cinnamon

Instructions

Preheat the oven to 375°F (190°C).

Cut the pears in half and remove the cores.

Place the pear halves in a baking dish, cut-side up.

Drizzle honey over each pear half and sprinkle with ground cinnamon.

Bake for 20-25 minutes or until the pears are tender.

Frozen Banana Popsicles:

Ingredients

Ripe bananas

Wooden popsicle sticks

Crushed nuts (e.g., almonds, pistachios)

Instructions

Peel the bananas and cut them in half.

Insert a wooden popsicle stick into each banana half.

Roll the bananas in crushed nuts.

Place the bananas on a baking sheet lined with parchment paper.

Freeze for a few hours until solid.

Mixed Fruit Sorbet:

Ingredients

Mixed frozen fruits (e.g., strawberries, mangoes, pineapples)

Fresh orange juice

Honey or agave syrup (optional)

Instructions

In a blender, combine the frozen fruits and fresh orange juice.

Blend until smooth and creamy.

Add honey or agave syrup if you want it sweeter.

Pour the sorbet into a container and freeze for a few hours before serving.

Almond Flour Banana Bread:

Ingredients

Ripe bananas

Almond flour

Eggs

Baking powder

Vanilla extract

Honey or maple syrup (optional)

Instructions

Preheat the oven to 350°F (175°C) and grease a loaf pan.

In a bowl, mash the ripe bananas.

Add almond flour, eggs, baking powder, vanilla extract, and sweetener if using.

Mix until well combined and pour the batter into the loaf pan.

Bake for about 45-50 minutes or until a toothpick inserted comes out clean.

Oatmeal Cookies:

Ingredients

Rolled oats

Whole wheat flour

Raisins

Chopped nuts (e.g., walnuts, pecans)

Coconut oil

Honey or maple syrup

Instructions

Preheat the oven to 350°F (175°C) and line a baking sheet with parchment paper.

In a bowl, mix rolled oats, whole wheat flour, raisins, and chopped nuts.

Add melted coconut oil and honey or maple syrup.

Stir until all ingredients are well combined.

Scoop tablespoonfuls of dough onto the baking sheet and flatten them slightly.

Bake for 12-15 minutes or until the edges turn golden brown.

Coconut Milk Rice Pudding:

Ingredients

Cooked brown rice

Coconut milk (full-fat or light)

Diced mango

Maple syrup or coconut sugar

Instructions

In a saucepan, combine cooked brown rice and coconut milk.

Bring to a simmer over low heat, stirring occasionally.

Add diced mango and sweeten with maple syrup or coconut sugar to taste.

Cook until the mixture thickens to a pudding-like consistency.

Baked Peaches:

Ingredients

Ripe peaches

Ricotta cheese

Honey

Ground cinnamon

Instructions

Preheat the oven to 375°F (190°C) and line a baking dish with parchment paper.

Cut the peaches in half and remove the pits.

Place the peach halves in the baking dish, cut-side up.

Fill each peach half with a spoonful of ricotta cheese.

Drizzle honey over the top and sprinkle with ground cinnamon.

Bake for 15-20 minutes or until the peaches are soft and slightly caramelized.

Orange and Pistachio Salad:

Ingredients

Oranges (peeled and sliced)

Pistachio nuts (shelled and chopped)

Fresh mint leaves

Instructions

Arrange the orange slices on a serving plate.

Sprinkle chopped pistachio nuts over the oranges.

Garnish with fresh mint leaves.

Quinoa and Mixed Berry Parfait:

Ingredients

Cooked quinoa

Mixed berries (e.g., blueberries, raspberries)

Greek yogurt

Honey or agave syrup

Instructions

In a glass or bowl, layer cooked quinoa, mixed berries, and Greek yogurt.

Drizzle honey or agave syrup for added sweetness.

Baked Apricots with Ricotta Cheese:

Ingredients

Fresh apricots

Ricotta cheese

Honey

Instructions

Preheat the oven to 375°F (190°C) and line a baking sheet with parchment paper.

Cut the apricots in half and remove the pits.

Place the apricot halves on the baking sheet, cut-side up.

Fill each apricot half with a spoonful of ricotta cheese.

Drizzle honey over the top.

Bake for 10-15 minutes or until the apricots are soft and slightly caramelized.

Lemon Chia Seed Muffins:

Ingredients

Chia seeds

Whole wheat flour

Baking powder

Lemon zest

Lemon juice

Eggs

Greek yogurt

Honey or maple syrup

Instructions

Preheat the oven to 350°F (175°C) and line a muffin tin with paper liners.

In a bowl, mix chia seeds, whole wheat flour, baking powder, and lemon zest.

In another bowl, whisk together lemon juice, eggs, Greek yogurt, and sweetener.

Combine the wet and dry ingredients, stirring until just combined.

Pour the batter into the muffin tin, filling each cup about 3/4 full.

Bake for 15-20 minutes or until a toothpick inserted comes out clean.

Kiwi and Strawberry Salsa:

Ingredients

Kiwi (peeled and diced)

Strawberries (diced)

Fresh mint leaves (chopped)

Instructions

In a bowl, combine diced kiwi and strawberries.

Add chopped fresh mint and mix well.

Serve with whole-grain crackers.

Baked Cinnamon Pita Chips:

Ingredients

Whole wheat pita bread

Coconut oil

Ground cinnamon

Instructions

Preheat the oven to 350°F (175°C) and line a baking sheet with parchment paper.

Cut the pita bread into triangles or squares.

Brush both sides of the pita pieces with melted coconut oil.

Sprinkle ground cinnamon over the pita chips.

Bake for 10-12 minutes or until the chips are crispy and golden.

Avocado Chocolate Mousse:

Ingredients

Ripe avocados

Cocoa powder

Almond milk

Maple syrup or honey

Instructions

In a blender or food processor, combine ripe avocados, cocoa powder, and almond milk.

Blend until smooth and creamy.

Sweeten with maple syrup or honey to taste.

Chill in the refrigerator before serving.

Blueberry and Oat Bars:

Ingredients

Rolled oats

Whole wheat flour

Blueberry filling (fresh or frozen blueberries with a touch of honey)

Coconut oil

Honey

Instructions

Preheat the oven to 350°F (175°C) and grease a baking dish.

In a bowl, mix rolled oats, whole wheat flour, and a drizzle of honey.

Add melted coconut oil and mix until the mixture becomes crumbly.

Press half of the mixture into the baking dish to form a crust.

Spread the blueberry filling over the crust.

Sprinkle the remaining oat mixture over the blueberry filling.

Bake for 30-35 minutes or until the top turns golden brown.

CHAPTER 5: FINAL THOUGHTS!

Finally, if you're concerned about the state of your heart throughout menopause, this cookbook is here to help. Hormonal shifts during perimenopause can have an effect on a woman's cardiovascular health, so it's important for her to make decisions that are good for her heart.

In this cookbook, we've covered a wide range of heart-healthy foods and nutritional guidelines developed with perimenopausal women in mind. Each dish has been carefully created to promote heart function without sacrificing taste or enjoyment, using nutrient-dense foods and creative culinary preparations.

Although a healthy diet is an important part of this cookbook there are other ways to take care of your heart as well. For optimal cardiovascular health, it is crucial to include exercise, stress reduction, and other heart-healthy habits into everyday living.

With the right information, you can take charge of your heart health during perimenopause and beyond. In this new phase of your life, you have the power to put your heart health first via the choices you make in what you eat and how you live.

Take this cookbook with you as you work toward a heart-healthy way of life. Savor the delicious and healthy dishes that honor your heart and well-being, and here's to thriving during perimenopause and beyond! We raise a glass to your eternal cardiovascular wellness.

Regular Monitoring and Heart Health Screening

In order to ensure the best possible cardiovascular health, regular monitoring and screening are needed. Early detection of possible cardiac problems can be achieved by regular monitoring of important health markers and tests. Hormonal changes throughout perimenopause and beyond can have an effect on cardiovascular health, making a preventative strategy all the more crucial at this time.

Blood pressure is a vital sign to track. Hypertension, often known as high blood pressure, is a leading cause of cardiovascular disease and strokes. Changes or anomalies in blood pressure can be detected with regular monitoring, either at home with a blood pressure monitor or at regular medical checkups. If high blood pressure is identified, it is possible to control it by diet, exercise, and, if required, medication.

Cholesterol levels are another important health indicator. Increased risk of atherosclerosis and cardiovascular disease is associated with both high levels of LDL cholesterol ("bad" cholesterol) and low levels of HDL cholesterol ("good" cholesterol). Cholesterol levels can be measured with a blood test, and recommendations for lifestyle modifications and medication, if necessary, can be made based on the results.

High blood sugar and diabetes put people at an increased risk of cardiovascular disease, making it all the more important to keep an eye on their blood sugar levels. Testing for diabetes and prediabetes with routine blood glucose and glycated hemoglobin (HbA1c) measurements can improve cardiovascular health.

Because of the hormonal changes that occur during perimenopause, it is especially important for women to keep a close eye on their weight if they are concerned about their cardiovascular health. Improving heart health and decreasing the risk of heart disease can be greatly aided by maintaining a healthy weight or working towards weight loss, if necessary.

In addition to routine checks, periodic screenings for heart disease are essential for catching problems in their earliest stages. Electrocardiograms (ECGs or EKGs), stress tests, echocardiograms, and coronary calcium scans are all examples of heart health screenings that may be recommended depending on an individual's age and risk factors. Screenings like this can evaluate cardiac function, spot anomalies, and yield useful information for managing cardiovascular health on an individual basis.

The best way for individuals to take care of their cardiovascular health and detect any underlying abnormalities early is to be proactive and dedicated to frequent monitoring and screening. As a result, they will be better able to make educated decisions about making positive changes to their lifestyle, accessing the necessary medical treatment, and establishing heart-healthy behaviors that will serve them well in the long run. In order to maintain cardiovascular health during perimenopause and beyond, it is important to visit your doctor often and talk openly about any concerns you may have.

Printed in Great Britain
by Amazon

42130974R00139